Intraperitoneal Therapy for Ovarian Cancer

David S. Alberts • Mary C. Clouser
Lisa M. Hess (Editors)

Intraperitoneal Therapy for Ovarian Cancer

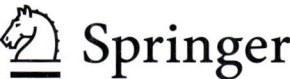 Springer

David S. Alberts
University of Arizona
College of Medicine
Arizona Cancer Center
1515 N. Campbell Ave.
Tucson, AZ 85724-5024
USA
dalberts@azcc.arizona.edu

Mary C. Clouser
University of Arizona
Arizona Cancer Center
1515 N. Campbell Ave.
Tucson, AZ 85724-5024
USA
mclouser@email.arizona.edu

Lisa M. Hess
Indiana University
School of Medicine
Departments of Public Health
and Obstetrics and Gynecology
714 N Senate Ave., EF250.
Indianapolis, IN 46202
lmhess@iupui.edu

ISBN: 978-3-642-12129-6   e-ISBN: 978-3-642-12130-2

DOI: 10.1007/978-3-642-12130-2

Springer Heidelberg Dordrecht London New York

Library of Congress Control Number: 2010925731

Cover design: eStudioCalamar, Figueres/Berlin

Printed on acid-free paper

Springer is part of Springer Science+Business Media (www.springer.com)

Acknowledgment

I have spent 40 years being devoted to the early detection and management of ovarian cancer. I have been amazed by the remarkable courage, grace, and beauty that our ovarian cancer survivors exhibit every day of their precious lives! This book is devoted to these social scientists, mothers, wives, and professionals who light up our lives with hope eternal that together we will conquer this heartbreaking disease! And, finally, to my magnificent wife, Heather, who through 50 years of a magnificent union and her own travail with breast cancer, "walks the talk" with loving compassion every day with her amazing Better Than Ever program to get women with cancer off the couch, out of the refrigerator, and into a healthful lifestyle.

Dave Alberts

Contents

Introduction

David S. Alberts and Setsuko K. Chambers

"While this research continues, however, we have a responsibility to ensure that women with advanced ovarian cancer who are candidates for IP therapy benefit from this treatment advance associated with such a remarkable improvement in overall survival [1]." This statement was printed in the January, 2006 National Cancer Institute's (NCI), Division of Cancer Treatment and Diagnosis announcement concerning the survival benefits of intraperitoneal chemotherapy for stage III ovarian cancer [1, 2]. Despite the efforts of the NCI, the Gynecologic Oncology Group (GOG), the Society for Gynecologic Oncology (SGO), and the American Society of Clinical Oncology (ASCO) to educate gynecologic and medical oncologists concerning the remarkable efficacy of intraperitoneal chemotherapy and the way it should be administered, the majority of women with stage III, optimally debulked disease, are not being offered or treated with intraperitoneal chemotherapy [3].

This lack of widespread use of intraperitoneal (IP) chemotherapy among today's oncologists has at its roots many causes, some more understandable than others. Certainly, the toxicities of early IP therapy that required intensive support and multiple interventions, coupled with catheter-related complications, dampened the initial enthusiasm. These critical, early negative experiences are understandably hard to overcome on an emotional level. However, our knowledge and skill have grown over three decades of IP therapy clinical trial research, and many of these challenges have now been overcome. Furthermore, the positive results of multiple randomized Phase III, NCI funded, nationally recognized, cooperative group clinical trials should by now have achieved standard of practice [4–6]. In a 2002 editorial in the *Journal of Clinical Oncology*, Drs. David Alberts, Maurie Markman, Deborah Armstrong, Mace Rothenberg, Franco Muggia, and Stephen Howell stated, "We cannot think of any other setting in oncology where the results of three positive phase III trials have not led to widespread adoption of the superior therapy. The time has come for IP chemotherapy to move beyond the setting of clinical trials and into the standard treatment armamentarium for women with optimally debulked stage III ovarian cancer. We owe our patients nothing less [7]." That being said, our task is to look forward, not backward, in terms of how we can prolong the lives of these extremely courageous women with advanced ovarian cancer who fight everyday to stay alive.

D.S. Alberts(✉) and S.K. Chambers
Director, Arizona Cancer Center, University of Arizona,
Tucson, AZ 85724-5024, USA
e-mail: dalberts@azcc.arizona.edu

D.S. Alberts et al. (eds.), *Intraperitoneal Therapy for Ovarian Cancer*,
DOI: 10.1007/978-3-642-12130-2_1, © Springer-Verlag Berlin Heidelberg 2010

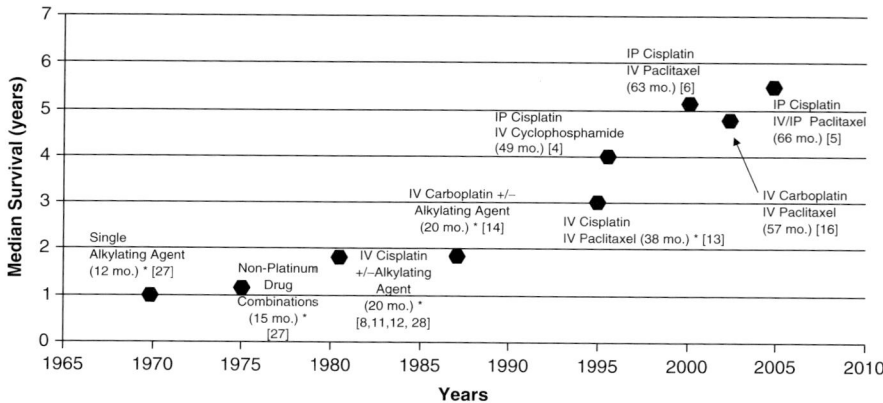

Fig. 1.1 Chronology of improvement in survival duration for advanced epithelial ovarian cancer focused on the development of intraperitoneal chemotherapy

While evaluating the chronology of treatment advances for advanced ovarian cancer, there have been a few seminal events during the last 40 years, as shown in Fig. 1.1 and described below.

1. Documentation that total abdominal hysterectomy with bilateral salpingo-oopherectomy (TAH-BSO), omentectomy, and debulking of tumor down to less than 1 cm sized residual in the intraperitoneal space are associated with improved survival in patients with stage III epithelial ovarian cancer [8–10].
2. Identification of intravenous cisplatin as a potentially curative and tolerable drug in the treatment of advanced epithelial ovarian cancer [11, 12].
3. Development of the intravenous combination of cisplatin plus paclitaxel to prolong survival in patients with suboptimally resected stage III and IV ovarian cancer [13].
4. Development of intravenous (IV) carboplatin and the combination of carboplatin plus IV paclitaxel as a less toxic but equally effective alternative to IV cisplatin and the combination of cisplatin plus paclitaxel [14–16].
5. Documentation in phase III clinical trials that intraperitoneal cisplatin, as compared to intravenous cisplatin with or without intravenous paclitaxel, prolongs survival in patients with stage III optimally resected ovarian cancer [4, 6].
6. Documentation that the addition of intraperitoneal paclitaxel to intraperitoneal cisplatin may further prolong progression-free survival and overall survival to more than 5 years, in comparison to intravenous platinum/taxane regimens [5, 17].
7. Evidence from phase II trials that intravenous bevacizumab is associated with unusually high objective response rates and enhanced progression-free survival in patients with platinum-resistant, recurrent ovarian cancer [18–21]. Although phase III trials of bevacizumab in patients with ovarian cancer are yet to be completed, they likely will document a major impact on patient survival.

There are multiple erroneous concepts that continue to mitigate against the universal incorporation of intraperitoneal chemotherapy administration for stage III, optimally resected ovarian cancer. All of these will be addressed in-depth in the following chapters of this text, which are authored by highly experienced investigators in this field. We believe that it is important to correct the misconceptions that continue to hinder treatment progress as follows:

Misconception #1: Intraperitoneal cisplatin chemotherapy inherently is too toxic for standard of care treatment. In at least one head-to-head comparison of IP to IV cisplatin at 100 mg/m², the patients treated in the IP phase III trial arm experienced significantly less leukopenia, neutropenia, tinnitus, clinical hearing loss, and neuropathic pain [4]. Only abdominal pain of relatively short duration (related to the mandated 2L IP fluid volumes) was more common in the IP group. In GOG 0172, there was clearly more acute toxicity in the IP trial arm; however, the IP-treated patients received 33% more cisplatin than did those on the IV trial arm [5]. Furthermore, IV paclitaxel in the IP-treatment arm was administered as a 24-h infusion (as compared to a 3-h infusion in the IV-treatment arm). These facts in large part explain the imbalanced acute toxicities of the IP therapy in this study. An in-depth quality of life evaluation using the Functional Assessment of Cancer Therapy (FACT-O) instrument revealed equivalent scores for the IV and IP-treated patient populations 1 year after planned chemotherapy completion [22]. Thus there is hardly a cogent argument to indict the GOG 0172 IP experimental arm as "too toxic for standard usage," especially in light of the documented 16-month increase in median survival associated with its use. Please refer to book Chap. 4 for in-depth discussions of these issues.

Misconception #2: The procedure for intraperitoneal chemotherapy is technically difficult, time-consuming, expensive, and requires in-patient care. The techniques involved in the administration of intraperitoneal cisplatin, paclitaxel, and several other anticancer agents (e.g., carboplatin, fluorodeoxyuridine, interferon-alpha) have been greatly improved over more than three decades. With laparoscopic placement of an intravenous type infusion port (as opposed to the commercially available intraperitoneal type infusion ports), the administration of intraperitoneal drugs has become a routine outpatient procedure, as described in detail in Chaps. 3,6, and 8. Granted, in general, medical oncology fellowship training in this disease area has traditionally been weak or nonexistent, leading to the relative lack of interactions between medical oncologists and gynecologic oncologists in the outpatient setting. This gap in training has further compounded the steep learning curve for optimal intraperitoneal therapy management. The NCI's Division of Cancer Treatment and Diagnosis sponsored a Clinical Announcement supporting intraperitoneal therapy and greatly heightened educational efforts that are required in fellowship programs, NCI-designated Comprehensive and Clinical Cancer Centers, as well as Community Clinical Oncology Program sites, concerning all aspects of the outpatient management in the setting of intraperitoneal therapy [1, 2]. In the Women's Cancers Pavilion at the Arizona Cancer Center, we have had a long-term interdisciplinary clinical research effort, led by Dr. Setsuko K. Chambers, Director of Gynecologic Oncology, and her gynecologic oncology colleagues, Drs. Kenneth Hatch and Janiel Cragun and medical oncologist colleagues (Drs. Ana Maria Lopez, Michael Bookman, and David Alberts) and multiple, specially trained research and clinical nursing staff. Without a "buy-in" from medical oncology and gynecologic oncology training programs to develop interdisciplinary participation in educational forums, ovarian cancer patients likely will be denied potentially lifesaving therapy. See Chaps. 5, 6, 7, and 8 for in-depth discussions of these issues.

Misconception #3: The designs of the three positive phase III trials comparing IP to IV therapy were flawed. According to the Center For Evidence Based Medicine, University of Oxford guidelines, the most convincing level of clinical trials evidence is a metaanalysis of well-designed, adequately powered, phase III studies [23]. Presently, there are three published metaanalyses, all of which have documented a pooled overall survival benefit to IP regimens (i.e., HR 0.79, 95% CI: 0.70–0.89) [1, 2, 24, 25]. The NCI-sponsored metaanalysis led to a rare NCI Clinical Announcement in January, 2006 [2]. Basically, all women with stage III, optimally debulked ovarian cancer should be educated about the potential benefits of cisplatin-based intraperitoneal therapy.

Virtually, all adequately powered phase III cancer clinical trials have design flaws, some large and some small. Ultimately, what counts is consistency in the results, as documented in the three IP vs. IV trial metaanalyses that have been published in *Gynecologic Oncology*, the *Cochrane Data Base of Systematic Reviews*, and *International Journal of Gynecologic Cancer* [1, 24, 25]. In Chap. 4 of this text there is a detailed discussion about the controversies involved in the pivotal phase III trial results (e.g., see Table 4.6).

Misconception 4: The future of intraperitoneal therapy is poor in the era of molecularly targeted drug development. Clearly, the landscape for molecularly targeted drug development for advanced ovarian cancer is expanding rapidly. It is extremely likely that the primary treatment of advanced ovarian cancer, whether optimally or suboptimally debulked, will change as the survival data from research protocol GOG 0218 (a phase III trial of IV carboplatin plus paclitaxel with or without bevacizumab) become available. The results of multiple phase II trials of bevacizumab in mainly platinum-resistant, recurrent disease have documented objective response rates of 15–25% (and 30–40% of patients progression-free at 6 months) with excellent tolerance [18, 21]. The initial concerns about relatively high rates of bowel perforation have diminished as larger safety analyses have been published [18, 21]. Of extreme relevance to both the continuing evaluation of intraperitoneal therapy and the role of intravenous bevacizumab is the activation of GOG 0252 (in the GOG), which will compare IV carboplatin plus IV paclitaxel (i.e., weekly regimen) to IP carboplatin plus weekly IV paclitaxel or IP cisplatin plus IV/IP paclitaxel. IV bevacizumab has been added to all three study arms, assuming that GOG 0218 will document a survival advantage for the bevacizumab in the phase III trial design [18, 26] (Walker 2009, Personal communication concerning Gynecologic Oncology Group protocol GOG 0252).

Obviously, bevacizumab has a major head start over other targeted agents for the management of advanced ovarian cancer; however, numerous other targeted agents are in earlier stages of development as discussed in Chaps. 7 and 9 of this text. With the explosion of drug development for advanced ovarian cancer, it will become more difficult to identify large numbers of eligible patient participants for any future, individual trial, unless we invite international research participation.

Misconception #5: There is no room for innovation to further improve intraperitoneal chemotherapy for advanced ovarian cancer. As discussed in Chaps. 8, 9, 10, and 11, there is tremendous opportunity for innovation in IP drug administration (e.g., selection of intra-peritoneal infusion solutions and improvement in IP drug delivery technology), the testing of novel cytotoxic drugs and biologic agents, further development of hyperthermic, intra-operative cytotoxic drug perfusions, and for improvement in supportive care procedures. In fact, we are just at the dawn of the era of the universal establishment of intraperitoneal therapy for advanced, surgically debulked ovarian cancer; however, for IP administration to be successful, it will take much greater outreach educational efforts at all levels of par-ticipants, including gynecologic oncologists, medical oncologists, oncology nurses, phar-macologists, and pharmacists, as well as the patients themselves. Ultimately, the national cooperative clinical trials groups, including the GOG and the Southwest Oncology Group (SWOG), with considerably more support from the NCI, must become dedicated in advancing this burgeoning field of drug discovery and research translation. Our patients deserve no less!

References

1. Trimble EL, Christian MC (2006) Intraperitoneal chemotherapy for women with advanced epithelial ovarian carcinoma. Gynecol Oncol 100(1):3–4
2. Trimble EL, Alvarez RD (2006) Intraperitoneal chemotherapy and the NCI clinical announce-ment. Gynecol Oncol 103(2 suppl 1):S18–S19
3. Rowan K (2009) Intraperitoneal therapy for ovarian cancer: why has it not become standard. JNCI 101(11):775–777
4. Alberts DS et al (1996) Intraperitoneal cisplatin plus intravenous cyclophosphamide versus intravenous cisplatin plus intravenous cyclophosphamide for stage III ovarian cancer. N Engl J Med 335(26):1950–1955
5. Armstrong DK et al (2006) Intraperitoneal cisplatin and paclitaxel in ovarian cancer. N Engl J Med 354(1):34–43
6. Markman M et al (2001) Phase III trial of standard-dose intravenous cisplatin plus paclitaxel versus moderately high-dose carboplatin followed by intravenous paclitaxel and intraperito-neal cisplatin in small-volume stage III ovarian carcinoma: an intergroup study of the Gynecologic Oncology Group, Southwestern Oncology Group, and Eastern Cooperative Oncology Group. J Clin Oncol 19(4):1001–1007
7. Alberts DS et al (2002) Intraperitoneal therapy for stage III ovarian cancer: a therapy whose time has come! J Clin Oncol 20(19):3944–3946
8. Bristow RE et al (2002) Survival effect of maximal cytoreductive surgery for advanced ovar-ian carcinoma during the platinum era: a meta-analysis. J Clin Oncol 20(5):1248–1259
9. Griffiths CT (1975) Surgical resection of tumor bulk in the primary treatment of ovarian car-cinoma. Natl Cancer Inst Monogr 42:101–104
10. Wharton JT, Herson J (1981) Surgery for common epithelial tumors of the ovary. Cancer 48 (2 Suppl):582–589
11. Thigpen JT et al (1983) Cis-platinum in the treatment of advanced or recurrent adenocarci-noma of the ovary. A phase II study of the Gynecologic Oncology Group. Am J Clin Oncol 6(4):431–435
12. Wiltshaw E, Kroner T (1976) Phase II study of cis-dichlorodiammineplatinum(II) (NSC-119875) in advanced adenocarcinoma of the ovary. Cancer Treat Rep 60(1):55–60
13. McGuire WP et al (1996) Cyclophosphamide and cisplatin compared with paclitaxel and cis-platin in patients with stage III and stage IV ovarian cancer. N Engl J Med 334(1):1–6

14. Alberts DS et al (1992) Improved therapeutic index of carboplatin plus cyclophosphamide versus cisplatin plus cyclophosphamide: final report by the Southwest Oncology Group of a phase III randomized trial in stages III and IV ovarian cancer. J Clin Oncol 10(5):706–717

15. Bookman MA et al (1996) Carboplatin and paclitaxel in ovarian carcinoma: a phase I study of the Gynecologic Oncology Group. J Clin Oncol 14(6):1895–1902

16. Ozols RF et al (2003) Phase III trial of carboplatin and paclitaxel compared with cisplatin and paclitaxel in patients with optimally resected stage III ovarian cancer: a Gynecologic Oncology Group study. J Clin Oncol 21(17):3194–3200

17. Rothenberg ML et al (2003) Combined intraperitoneal and intravenous chemotherapy for women with optimally debulked ovarian cancer: results from an intergroup phase II trial. J Clin Oncol 21(7):1313–1319

18. Burger RA et al (2007) Phase II trial of bevacizumab in persistent or recurrent epithelial ovarian cancer or primary peritoneal cancer: a Gynecologic Oncology Group Study. J Clin Oncol 25(33):5165–5171

19. Cannistra SA et al (2007) Phase II study of bevacizumab in patients with platinum-resistant ovarian cancer or peritoneal serous cancer. J Clin Oncol 25(33):5180–5186

20. Chura JC et al (2007) Bevacizumab plus cyclophosphamide in heavily pretreated patients with recurrent ovarian cancer. Gynecol Oncol 107:326–330

21. Garcia AA et al (2008) Phase II clinical trial of bevacizumab and low-dose metronomic oral cyclophosphamide in recurrent ovarian cancer: a trial of the California, Chicago, and Princess Margaret Hospital phase II consortia. J Clin Oncol 26(1):76–82

22. Wenzel LB et al (2007) Health-related quality of life during and after intraperitoneal versus intravenous chemotherapy for optimally debulked ovarian cancer: a Gynecologic Oncology Group Study. J Clin Oncol 25(4):437–443

23. Phillips B et al (2009) Oxford Centre for Evidence-based Medicine Levels of Evidence. [Cited; Available from: http://www.cebm.net/index]

24. Hess LM et al (2007) A meta-analysis of the efficacy of intraperitoneal cisplatin for the frontline treatment of ovarian cancer. Int J Gynecol Cancer 17(3):561–570

25. Jaaback K, Johnson N (2006) Intraperitoneal chemotherapy for the initial management of primary epithelial ovarian cancer (review), in Cochrane database of systematic reviews. Wiley, New York

26. McMeekin DD et al (2009) Phase II study of intravenous (IV) bevacizumab and paclitaxel, and intraperitoneal (IP) cisplatin, followed by bevacizumab consolidation for advanced ovarian (O) or peritoneal (P) cancers. J Clin Oncol 27(suppl; abstr 5540):15s

27. Omura GA et al (1983) A randomized comparison of melphalan versus melphalan plus hexamethylmelamine versus adriamycin plus cyclophosphamide in ovarian carcinoma. Cancer 51(5):783–789

28. Omura G et al (1986) A randomized trial of cyclophosphamide and doxorubicin with or without cisplatin in advanced ovarian carcinoma. A Gynecologic Oncology Group Study. Cancer 57(9):1725–1730

Current Chemotherapy of Ovarian Cancer

2

Michael A Bookman

2.1
Trials that Define Primary Treatment

Current optimal management of advanced-stage ovarian cancer includes maximal cytoreductive surgery and a program of chemotherapy with carboplatin and paclitaxel, generally administered for six cycles. While the chemotherapy has been validated by phase III trials, there are areas of controversy, as well as gaps in knowledge, contributing to acceptable variations in clinical practice as applied to individual patients. A number of strategies have been evaluated with the goal of improving treatment outcomes, including dose intensity, maintenance-consolidation, schedule variations, intraperitoneal administration, regional hyperthermia, and incorporation of additional cytotoxic agents. Many of the phase III trials that have defined current treatment options are summarized in Table 2.1.

Platinum compounds remain dominant as the most active cytotoxic agents currently utilized in the treatment of ovarian cancer. Over the last 30 years, the therapeutic ratio of platinum-based primary chemotherapy has been improved through the development of less toxic analogs (carboplatin) and the determination of optimal dose, schedule, sequence, and duration of treatment [1–4]. In general, the administration of higher doses of chemotherapy with hematopoietic support, or extended administration of multiple cycles of chemotherapy (beyond six cycles), has not improved long-term outcomes, and these strategies carry an increased risk of serious cumulative toxicity [5–7].

M.A. Bookman
Arizona Cancer Center, 1515 N. Campbell Avenue, 2942F,
P.O. Box 245024,Tucson, AZ 85724-5024, USA
e-mail: mbookman@azcc.arizona.edu

D.S. Alberts et al. (eds.), *Intraperitoneal Therapy for Ovarian Cancer*,
DOI: 10.1007/978-3-642-12130-2_2, © Springer-Verlag Berlin Heidelberg 2010

Table 2.1 Principles of optimal primary therapy

Platinum agents	Cisplatin vs. carboplatin	Carboplatin dosing optimized using renal clearance [2] Carboplatin-based combinations associated with equivalent long-term outcomes, reduced nonhematologic toxicity, and increased hematologic toxicity, especially thrombocytopenia [1, 3, 4]
	Carboplatin dose intensity	No evidence of improved long-term outcomes within ranges achieved using conventional therapy or hematopoietic progenitor cell support [5–7]
	Duration of treatment	Optimal number of cycles not defined, without differences in long-term outcomes between 4, 6, 8, 10, or 12 cycles within individual trials. Cumulative hematologic and nonhematologic toxicity observed with extended therapy, and most patients receive six cycles
Taxanes	Dose intensity and infusion duration	No evidence for dose-response relationship within practical dose range [76–78] Extended infusion duration correlates with hematologic toxicity, but not efficacy [79, 80]
	Primary combinations with cisplatin or carboplatin	Improved median survival with paclitaxel and platinum [8–10] "Platelet-sparing effect" in combination with carboplatin raises questions of drug–drug antagonism [28] Sequential single-agent therapy appropriate for some patients [12, 13]
	Optimal scheduling	Improved therapeutic ratio (phase I-II) associated with weekly therapy in recurrent disease [16, 17] Improved progression-free survival with dose-dense weekly paclitaxel in combination with carboplatin as primary treatment [18]
	Docetaxel vs. paclitaxel	Different toxicity profile without improved long-term outcomes [15]
Intraperitoneal therapy	Intraperitoneal cisplatin	Improved survival validated in phase III trials, but with increased nonhematologic toxicity [81–83] Metaanalysis [84, 85] Commentary [86, 87]
	Intraperitoneal carboplatin	Reduction in nonhematologic toxicity, but activated more slowly, compared to cisplatin. Potential role as intraperitoneal therapy currently under phase III evaluation (GOG 0252)
	Intraperitoneal paclitaxel	Incorporated as component in GOG 0172, but individual contribution of route vs. schedule unclear [82]

Table 2.1 (continued)

Incorporation of additional agents with primary therapy	Integration of cytotoxic agents including gemcitabine, epirubicin, PEG-liposomal doxorubicin, topotecan	Extensively evaluated through international phase III trials involving multiple GCIG members. No evidence for improved progression-free or overall survival with any new regimen [22–26]
	Integration of agents that target angiogenesis	Positive phase II data with single-agent bevacizumab, front-line phase III trials ongoing (GOG 0218, OV7) [50, 51]
Maintenance – consolidation	Extended cytotoxic therapy evaluated with topotecan, epirubicin, paclitaxel, or IP platinum	No improvement in survival from completed trials [88–92]. Phase III trial in progress with paclitaxel and polyglutamated paclitaxel (GOG 0212)
	Extended biologic therapy evaluated with interferon-α, [46]Y-anti-HMFG1 antibody, murine anti-CA125	No improvement in survival from completed trials [93–95]. Trials in progress with anti-MUC16 antibody, bevacizumab, and inhibitors of VEGF receptor signaling
Surgical interventions	Extent of cytoreductive surgery	Extent of postoperative residual disease correlated with outcome in retrospective studies, although cytoreductive surgery has not been prospectively validated in a randomized trial [96–98]
	Timing of cytoreductive surgery	Initial surgery followed by interval cytoreduction in appropriate patients is not inferior to initial cytoreduction alone [99–101] For patients with advanced IIIC-IV disease, neoadjuvant chemotherapy with interval cytoreduction achieves equivalent survival to initial cytoreduction, with improved safety (EORTC 55971)
	Role of secondary surgical assessment	Secondary surgical assessment for patients in clinical complete remission provides prognostic information, but surgery has not been shown to have an impact on survival or optimization of secondary treatment [102]

2.2
Optimal Integration of Taxanes

Mature results from Gynecologic Oncology Group (GOG) protocol GOG 0111 and the National Cancer Institute of Canada (NCIC) and European Organization for Research and Treatment of Cancer (EORTC) trial, protocol OV10, established the superiority of cisplatin plus paclitaxel as compared to cisplatin plus cyclophosphamide [8–10]. In addition, GOG 0158 and Abeitsgemeinschaft Gynäkologische Onkologie-Ovarialkarzinom

(Gynecologic Oncology Ovarian Cancer Study Group, AGO-OVAR) studies established that carboplatin plus paclitaxel was at least as effective as cisplatin plus paclitaxel [3, 4]. Based on these findings, the Gynecologic Cancer InterGroup (GCIG) published consensus guidelines favoring carboplatin and paclitaxel as the preferred comparator arm for clinical trials [11]. However, the GOG 0132 and International Collaborative Ovarian Neoplasm (ICON3) trials have suggested that sequential therapy with platinum followed by paclitaxel at progression can achieve equivalent long-term outcomes for some patients, supporting a role for individualized selection criteria while reinforcing the primary activity of platinum compounds [12, 13].

Taxanes have clearly emerged as the second most important class of cytotoxic agents. In addition to data from front-line trials, a phase III trial in the setting of platinum-sensitive recurrent disease, ICON4, also demonstrated superiority of a combination of carboplatin and paclitaxel compared to carboplatin regimens without paclitaxel, but without directly addressing the role of sequential single-agent therapy [14].

Substitution of docetaxel is an acceptable alternative to paclitaxel in the front-line setting with a reduced risk of neuropathy and hypersensitivity, but with an increased risk of dose-limiting hematologic toxicity, based on a phase III trial [15]. In spite of interesting molecular pharmacodynamics, there are no data to indicate clinical superiority of docetaxel when compared to paclitaxel in the management of newly diagnosed or recurrent epithelial ovarian cancer.

With paclitaxel, longer infusions ($\geq$24 h) increase mucosal and bone marrow toxicity, but without improved efficacy. Shorter infusions (<3 h) are generally better-tolerated from a hematologic perspective, although higher individual doses can increase the risk of arthralgia-myalgia and neuropathy. Weekly scheduling permits higher cumulative dose delivery, while avoiding hematologic toxicity and alopecia, and has demonstrated consistent activity in patients who have recurred within 6 months of primary therapy with conventional carboplatin and paclitaxel [16, 17].

The Japanese Gynecologic Oncology Group (JGOG) conducted a phase III trial in women with newly diagnosed advanced-stage ovarian cancer, demonstrating superiority of weekly dose-dense paclitaxel in combination with standard doses of carboplatin compared to standard scheduling of the same drugs [18]. This is an important finding, illustrating the need to carefully examine how we use standard agents, as well as strategies to incorporate new agents. Ongoing phase III trials through GOG and other groups aim to extend the JGOG findings, including integration with intraperitoneal chemotherapy and bevacizumab.

2.3
Integration of a Third Cytotoxic Agent

A number of nonplatinum cytotoxic agents have well-defined activity in the management of recurrent disease, including topotecan, pegylated liposomal doxorubicin (PLD), prolonged oral etoposide, and gemcitabine. Each of these agents has a unique molecular target, mechanism of action, and pathways of resistance. In view of the central role of platinum, there has been particular interest in the incorporation of agents that may accentuate the platinum response, through increased formation of platinum-deoxyribonucleic acid (DNA) adducts or inhibition of DNA repair. Early nonrandomized clinical trials reported high response rates using triple-drug platinum-based combinations, particularly with gemcitabine [19, 20]. However, randomized studies were clearly needed to determine whether new platinum-based combinations could achieve meaningful clinical benefit when balanced against the increased risk of host toxicity.

Recognizing that a large number of patients would be required for a definitive analysis of newer cytotoxic agents, many of the cooperative groups engaged in collaborative relationships through GCIG, which provided a framework for sharing preliminary clinical data, coordinated planning of international phase III trials and standards for collaboration on larger studies [21]. While some international trials emerged with overlapping treatment regimens, the cumulative global experience provides a robust analysis of multiple platinum-based chemotherapy regimens for primary therapy of advanced-stage disease.

Based on multiple phase III trials involving more than ten thousand women, we can conclude that the addition of a third cytotoxic agent has clearly been associated with increased host toxicity, but has not been shown to improve long-term clinical outcomes [22–26]. Some agents, such as topotecan and gemcitabine, exhibit schedule- and sequence-dependent hematologic toxicity, particularly when combined with carboplatin. These agents can interfere with repair of damage from platinum-DNA adducts, which could be advantageous, but only if there was a reliable method to circumvent hematologic toxicity. Of note, the relationship between increased hematologic toxicity and optimum tumor cell-kill has remained unclear, and one may not always correlate with the other [27].

In contrast, combinations of paclitaxel with carboplatin are well-tolerated, with capability of administering full doses of both drugs. This has been attributed to a "platelet-sparing" effect of paclitaxel on carboplatin-mediated thrombocytopenia, raising questions about possible drug–drug antagonism which have not been resolved [28].

2.4
New Approaches Targeting the Mitotic Apparatus

Disruption of the mitotic apparatus is thought to be the primary mechanism of action for paclitaxel, which promotes tubulin aggregation. The clinical development of paclitaxel has been challenged by poor solubility, hypersensitivity reactions, and peripheral neuropathy. Various formulations have been developed to optimize delivery, including liposomes, nanoparticle albumin-bound (NAB) paclitaxel, polyglutamated paclitaxel, and emulsions. NAB-paclitaxel has regulatory approval for the treatment of metastatic breast cancer and phase II activity in ovarian cancer [29]. While a front-line phase III trial of NAB-paclitaxel in combination with carboplatin would be of interest, there are many competing priorities, including novel cytotoxic and molecular-targeted agents, as well as the utilization of non-conjugated paclitaxel on a dose-dense weekly schedule.

Alternative agents under development include potent epothilone derivatives (ixabepilone and patupilone) that also target tubulin, but are less susceptible to some resistance strategies, such as increased expression of tubulin beta-III isoforms or multidrug resistance (MDR) mediated by p-glycoprotein (pGP) [30]. These agents are associated with varying degrees of myelosuppression, stomatitis, diarrhea, and neuropathy. Another approach has been to develop molecules that inhibit proteins associated with the mitotic spindle apparatus, including the kinesin spindle protein (KSP). These agents, if proven to be effective, would eliminate the risk of neuropathy, which is caused by damage to nonmitotic tubulin. There has also been interest in targeting aurora kinase, which is frequently overexpressed in tumors and associated with regulation of chromosome segregation and cytokinesis during mitosis.

2.5
Development of Alternative Cytotoxic Agents

While the combination of carboplatin and paclitaxel remains a well-tolerated and effective standard treatment for newly diagnosed ovarian cancer, there is continued interest in the discovery of new targets, as well as new approaches for inhibiting old targets. DNA damage, replication, and repair offer a number of important targets for ongoing drug development. For example, trabectedin, a marine-derived antineoplastic agent, was initially isolated from the tunicate Ecteinascidia turbinata. It binds covalently to the minor groove of DNA, bending DNA toward the major groove, disrupting transcription, and leading to G2-M cell cycle arrest and apoptosis. Trabectedin is particularly active in recurrent platinum-sensitive ovarian cancer [31]. However, unlike carboplatin, trabectedin is more cytotoxic in cells with efficient transcription-coupled nucleotide excision repair (NER).

Folate metabolism is another pathway under reexamination, with the development of pemetrexed, a multitargeted antifolate that is also an excellent substrate for polyglutamation, thereby increasing retention within tumor cells. Pemetrexed, in combination with cisplatin, is utilized for the treatment of mesothelioma, and single-agent pemetrexed has activity in recurrent platinum-resistant ovarian cancer, with expected hematologic toxicity managed with dose selection and utilization of vitamin supplementation [32, 33].

Although there is great interest in molecular-targeted biology, cytotoxic chemotherapy remains an essential element in the treatment of advanced-stage disease. New cytotoxic agents with novel targets should be fully evaluated in parallel with biologic agents.

2.6
Biologic Principles with an Impact on Primary Therapy

Primary disease management has been guided not only by phase III trials, but also by emerging knowledge of cancer biology, including histopathology. For example, although primary ovarian mucinous tumors are rare, collaborative retrospective review of international data has verified that mucinous tumors are not generally responsive to platinum-based chemotherapy, and patients with advanced mucinous tumors have inferior long-term survival, compared with serous or endometrioid subtypes [34, 35]. International studies have been initiated through the GCIG to evaluate alternative interventions, modeled after mucinous colorectal cancer (Table 2.2).

Table 2.2 Biologic observations guiding development of front-line trials

Type I/II tumors	Clinical and molecular characteristics of low-grade (type I) and high-grade serous tumors (type II)	Verified distinct origin of low-grade serous tumors in association with borderline tumors of low malignant potential, compared to high-grade serous tumors, reinforcing targeted development of clinical trials [39, 40]
Early-stage disease	Clinical features, pathologic subtypes, and risk factors associated with early-stage disease	Recognition of distinct distribution of histologic subtypes in early-stage disease, relationship of complete surgical staging to chemotherapy outcomes, risk of recurrence associated with high-grade serous histology and/or positive peritoneal cytology, reduced risk associated with well-staged clear cell tumors [36–38]
Advanced-stage disease	Analysis of histologic factors, molecular subtypes, and activated pathways	Verification that mucinous tumors are poorly-responsive to platinum-based therapy with inferior long-term clinical outcomes [34, 35] Identification of epithelial-mesenchymal transition, including mesenchymal gene activation profile with more aggressive behavior [44, 45]
Stem cell hypothesis	Presence of treatment-resistant regenerative subpopulations	Recognition of limitations associated with platinum-based primary therapy and the need to explore alternatives guided by molecular and genomic analysis of treatment-resistant subpopulations [61, 62]
Synthetic lethal paradigms	Genetic and epigenetic silencing of pathways involved in DNA repair	Opportunity to exploit synthetic lethality using PARP inhibition (± chemotherapy) in tumors with loss of BRCA function and deficient homologous recombination repair of double-strand DNA breaks [70, 71] Somatic and epigenetic silencing of BRCA, expanding the proportion of patients that might benefit from PARP inhibition [72, 73] Recognition of secondary mutations in BRCA associated with PARP resistance [74, 75]
Immunologic regulation	Intratumoral T lymphocytes	Improved survival associated with higher number of tumor infiltrating lymphocytes and lower ratios of immunoregulatory T lymphocytes, prompting prospective trials with vaccination, antibodies, and cytokines [103, 104]
Drug resistance	Platinum-resistance	Multifactorial, including transport, detoxification, damage tolerance, reduced damage detection, defective apoptotic signaling [55–57, 60]
	Multidrug resistance	Drug efflux pumps (p-glycoprotein) for natural products, no therapeutic advantage from inhibition [64]
	Other specific adaptations	Examples include isoforms of β tubulin associated with taxane resistance, downregulation of targets (topoisomerase I), reduced phosphorylation of gemcitabine, amplification of ribonucleotide reductase

It is also apparent that early-stage ovarian cancer has a distinct biologic profile, characterized by an increased proportion of nonserous tumors, including endometrioid and clear cell histology [36–38]. When patients undergo complete surgical staging and have a tumor that is limited to the ovary, the finding of clear cell histology, in and of itself, does not appear to carry an independent adverse prognosis, and cure would be expected in the vast majority of cases. In contrast, early-stage serous tumors are often high-grade and more likely to have occult peritoneal or nodal spread. As such, they have a greater risk of recurrence and are perhaps more likely to benefit from adjuvant chemotherapy.

In advanced-stage serous tumors, distinct molecular profiles have been associated with low-grade (Type I) compared to high-grade (Type II) neoplasia [39, 40]. Low-grade invasive adenocarcinoma generally arises in conjunction with borderline tumors of low malignant potential. These tumors are not generally sensitive to platinum-based chemotherapy, retain functional p53, and harbor activating mutations of either B-ras or K-raf [39, 40]. Activated RAS triggers phosphorylation and activation of RAF kinase, which then phosphorylates cytoplasmic mitogen-activated protein kinases (MAPK) that include MEK-1/2 [41]. Activated MEK then phosphorylates ERK-1/2, which dimerizes and translocates to the nucleus where it can regulate cellular proliferation [42]. This important pathway is activated by a diverse group of extracellular signals including integrins, receptors for epidermal growth factor, platelet-derived growth factor, and insulin-like growth factor-1, as well as various cytokines. Specific tyrosine kinase inhibitors, such as AZD6244, have been developed to target MEK-1/2, a central pathway component [43]. The GOG completed a phase II study of AZD6244, a MEK inhibitor, in low-grade ovarian adenocarcinoma (GOG 0239), and this may provide an important strategy to build new combinations.

In contrast, high-grade serous tumors tend to have inactivation of p53 through chromosomal deletion and/or mutation, without activating mutations of B-raf or K-ras, and are initially sensitive to platinum-based chemotherapy [39, 40]. Some high-grade ovarian cancers are associated with sarcomatous differentiation, recognized as carcinosarcomas or mixed Müllerian tumors. This is thought to occur through a process of epithelial-mesenchymal transition (EMT) and is associated with downregulation of epithelial markers (such as epithelial membrane antigen) and upregulation of mesenchymal markers (such as vimentin) [44]. These changes contribute to cellular motility, production of proteolytic enzymes, and invasive behavior. Aggressive mesenchymal features have also been identified through the analysis of gene expression profiles, even without visible evidence of sarcoma [45]. Core components of EMT are under control of src kinase, prompting clinical evaluation of dasatinib and other inhibitors of src kinase.

Advanced-stage clear cell tumors exhibit more aggressive patterns of metastatic spread and are frequently resistant to platinum-based chemotherapy. Analysis of gene expression profiles have identified characteristic patterns associated with clear cell tumors from other primary sites, but optimal treatment strategies for clear cell tumors of ovarian origin remain to be defined [46].

2.7
Targeting Angiogenesis

High-grade serous ovarian cancer is characterized by overexpression of vascular endothelial growth factor (VEGF), which drives abnormal tumor angiogenesis, contributing to high interstitial pressure and production of ascites [47]. Direct targeting of this pathway can be achieved by sequestration of VEGF protein using monoclonal antibodies (bevacizumab) or engineered binding site molecules (aflibercept), blockade of the VEGF receptor-2 (VEGFR2) with monoclonal antibodies (IMC-1C11), or inhibition of receptor-associated tyrosine kinase with small molecular weight inhibitors (axitinib, cediranib, pazopanib, sorafenib, BIBF 1120). Indirect strategies include targeting genes involved in the regulation of VEGF expression, such as hypoxia inducible factor 1-alpha (HIF1a), antibody-based blockade of angiopoietin-2 (CVX-060), inhibition of cytoplasmic tyrosine kinases that are activated following VEGF receptor-mediated phosphorylation, inhibition of protein kinase-c β (enzastaurin), or interference with other convergence pathways, such as the serine-threonine specific protein kinase (AKT) or the mammalian target of rapamycin (mTOR) [48, 49].

Thus far, the most widely studied agent has been bevacizumab, initially as a single agent, and subsequently in phase III trials with concurrent chemotherapy and maintenance [50, 51]. When evaluated in combination with chemotherapy in other tumor types, bevacizumab was associated with improved long-term outcomes, achieving regulatory approval in colon cancer, nonsquamous lung cancer, and breast cancer. These observations have been attributed to improved drug delivery as a result of pseudonormalization of tumor vasculature and a reduction in interstitial pressure [52]. Single-agent activity with bevacizumab in recurrent ovarian cancer is more substantial than previously observed in these other tumor types, and it is anticipated that combinations of bevacizumab with carboplatin and paclitaxel will improve long-term outcomes for women with ovarian cancer. These combinations are currently under evaluation in several phase III trials, both in the setting of primary therapy for newly diagnosed disease (GOG 0218, ICON7), as well as recurrent disease (GOG 0213).

2.8
Chemotherapy Resistance

The dominant pattern of resistance observed in ovarian cancer is related to platinum compounds (cisplatin and carboplatin), with extension to traditional alkylating agents and radiation [53, 54]. Resistance is multifactorial, involving decreased active transport, increased drug efflux, rapid detoxification of platinum through glutathione conjugation, increased DNA damage tolerance, reduced detection of DNA damage, accelerated removal of platinum-DNA adducts, enhanced DNA repair, and defective apoptotic signaling, often associated with loss of tumor suppressor protein p53, but also independent of p53. Resistance can be intrinsic or evolve in response to selective pressures from chemotherapy exposure. As such, some components of resistance may be reversible over a period of time.

Preclinical models have suggested a variety of strategies to prevent or overcome resistance. Frequently, these models are based on targeting one aspect of platinum-resistance using short-term data from established cell lines, and they have not successfully translated to clinical practice. Actual human tumors have lower growth fractions, greater biologic heterogeneity, and diverse adaptation strategies.

Currently, there are no compounds with the ability to specifically target platinum-resistant tumors in the clinical setting. Some chemotherapy agents, such as gemcitabine and topotecan, can interfere with DNA repair and reliably increase platinum-mediated toxicity. However, these effects are not tumor-specific, and combinations are also associated with increased hematologic toxicity, limiting their clinical application. A sterically-hindered platinum compound (picoplatin) was developed to avoid thiol-mediated inactivation, but did not achieve superior clinical outcomes in patients with recurrent disease [55]. It was also thought that oxaliplatin might retain activity in resistant tumors because it forms DNA adducts that are not detected by the mismatch repair system, but only a 7% response rate was observed in patients with a platinum-free interval of less than 6 months [56]. In addition, components of the mismatch repair system, such as MLH1, can be suppressed by gene methylation in resistant tumors, prompting studies with a demethylating agent (decitabine) and carboplatin, but without improved efficacy at the expense of increased hematologic toxicity [57].

NER is the primary mechanism to remove platinum-DNA adducts, and excision repair cross-complementing-1 (ERCC1) is a critical NER component. Resistance to platinum has been linked to ERCC1 mRNA expression in ovarian cancer and other tumors, and ERCC1 levels are predictive of clinical outcomes in lung cancer patients treated with platinum-based chemotherapy [58, 59]. Whether ERCC1, or other markers, could be used to guide chemotherapy selection in woman with ovarian cancer is unknown.

Recent efforts have focused on the biology of platinum influx, largely mediated by copper transporter-1 (CTR1), which can be downregulated after platinum exposure [60]. Strategies are also under evaluation to restore damage detection and apoptotic signaling in tumor cells via intrinsic or extrinsic pathways, such as restoration of the tumor suppressor gene protein p53, regulation of the antiapoptotic protein Bcl-2, activation of the tumor necrosis factor receptor (TNFR), and TNF-related apoptosis-inducing ligand (TRAIL) R1. There has also been interest in tumor stem cell biology as it relates to the emergence of drug resistant populations, and this may provide some new molecular markers and targets with greater specificity [61, 62].

The second pattern is related to MDR for natural products mediated primarily by the drug efflux pump, pGP. Natural substrates for pGP include taxanes, anthracyclines, and vinca alkaloids. A number of inhibitors of pGP MDR function have been developed [63]. The most extensively studied agent has been valspodar, an analog of cyclopsorine A, which showed no clinical benefit in a phase III trial with paclitaxel and carboplatin [64]. While these agents can block drug efflux at the cellular level, the effects are not tumor-specific, and it has been necessary to utilize lower doses of chemotherapy to avoid serious toxicity, minimizing any potential therapeutic advantage. The breast cancer resistance protein (BCRP), or adenosine triphosphate (ATP)-binding cassette protein G2 (ABCG2), dimerizes to form a membrane-associated energy-dependent efflux pump that is also associated with MDR, primarily to mitoxantrone and camptothecins, including topotecan [65].

The third pattern represents a collection of specific cellular adaptations associated with resistance to individual cytotoxic agents used in the treatment of ovarian cancer. These include mutations in β tubulin subunits or alterations in the ratio of tubulin isoforms that have an impact on taxane sensitivity. Downregulation of topoisomerase-I can prevent the formation of cleavable complexes with topotecan. Resistance to gemcitabine can be mediated by decreased active membrane transport, reduced phosphorylation related to the depletion of deoxycytidine kinase, or amplification of the gene for the M2 subunit of ribonucleotide reductase [66–68].

Our understanding of the biology surrounding drug resistance continues to improve, with interesting predictive markers of tumor response, and potential targets for intervention, but drug resistance still remains a central problem in the treatment of advanced-stage ovarian cancer.

2.9
Synthetic Lethal Strategies

Poly(adenosine diphosphate [ADP]-ribose) polymerase (PARP) is a key component in the process of base excision repair of single-strand DNA breaks. Inhibition of PARP leads to the accumulation of DNA single-strand breaks, which can lead to potentially lethal DNA double-strand breaks at replication forks [69]. However, these breaks are usually repaired by the double-strand homologous recombination pathway, which incorporates the tumor suppressor proteins BRCA1 and BRCA2. Germ-line mutations in either BRCA1 or BRCA2 have been associated with an increased risk of developing ovarian cancer, and tumor cells that harbor loss-of-function BRCA mutations (affecting the remaining wild-type allele) are deficient in homologous repair. Importantly, this repair defect is not shared by normal tissues in the same patient, due to the presence of the remaining wild-type allele.

Inhibition of PARP in a patient with a BRCA1/2 mutation has the potential to create a "synthetic lethal" situation, generating unrepaired single-strand breaks, accumulation of double-strand breaks, and collapse of the replication fork. This single-agent treatment strategy is well-tolerated and effective in a proportion of women with BRCA1/2 mutations [70, 71]. However, inheritable germ-line mutations only account for perhaps 5% of all ovarian cancers. Additional patients may benefit if they have tumors with somatic (non-germ line) mutations or with hypermethylation or epigenetic silencing of key genes involved in DNA homologous recombination repair [72, 73]. Allowing for all three scenarios might account for 30% of women with ovarian cancer. Of interest, laboratory studies have documented the appearance of secondary mutations in tumor-associated BRCA1 that can restore expression and overcome the effects of PARP inhibition [74, 75].

PARP inhibitors (olaparib, ABT-881, BSI-201) can also be utilized to enhance the effects of cytotoxic chemotherapeutics that target DNA, such as carboplatin, gemcitabine, and topotecan. However, as with other strategies to overcome drug resistance, there can be increased host toxicity, particularly bone marrow suppression, and randomized trials will be needed to evaluate long-term clinical benefits.

2.10
Discussion

Optimal primary chemotherapy of advanced ovarian cancer has not substantially changed over the last few years, in spite of the extensive evaluation of new cytotoxic agents and diverse treatment strategies (Table 2.3). Almost all patients undergo at least one attempt at

Table 2.3 Clinical impact of strategies to improve outcomes in primary therapy

Clinical paradigm and representative trials	Stage	Patients (n)	Hazard ratio for progression-free survival (95% CI)	p Value
Substitution of docetaxel for paclitaxel (SCOTROC) [15]	Ic–IV	1,077		
Paclitaxel + Carboplatin		538	1.0 (reference)	
Docetaxel + Carboplatin		539	0.97 (0.83–1.13)	p=0.707
Incorporation of a third cytotoxic agent (i.e GOG 0182/ICON5) [22]	III–IV	4,312		
Paclitaxel + Carboplatin		864	1.0 (reference)	
Gemcitabine triplet		864	1.028 (0.924–1.143)	p=0.610
Gemcitabine doublet		861	1.037 (0.932–1.153)	p=0.503
PEG-liposomal doxorubicin		862	0.984 (0.884–1.095)	p=0.796
Topotecan doublet		861	1.066 (0.958–1.186)	p=0.239
Intraperitoneal chemotherapy (GOG 0172) [82]	Optimal III	415		
Intravenous		210	1.0 (reference)	
Intraperitoneal		205	0.80 (0.64–1.00)	p=0.05
Dose-dense weekly paclitaxel with carboplatin (JGOG) [18]	II–IV	631		
Standard paclitaxel		319	1.0 (reference)	
Dose-dense paclitaxel		312	0.71 (0.58–0.88)	p=0.0015
Incorporation of bevacizumab				
GOG 0218	III–IV	1,873	Accrual complete, analysis in progress	
MRC-ICON7	Ic–IV	1,528	Accrual complete, analysis in progress	

maximal cytoreductive surgery, and the combination of carboplatin and paclitaxel remains a well-tolerated and widely utilized standard treatment regimen. Emerging data favor the selected utilization of neoadjuvant chemotherapy in patients with bulky disease, and dose-dense weekly paclitaxel in combination with carboplatin appears superior to standard dosing of paclitaxel. Intraperitoneal cisplatin and paclitaxel can be administered to patients with small-volume residual disease, and new trials are evaluating intraperitoneal delivery of carboplatin to improve patient safety and tolerability.

The integration of emerging biologic principles with the development of molecular-targeted reagents is starting to achieve meaningful results, especially with regard to inhibition of angiogenesis and interference with PARP-mediated DNA repair. Biologic observations have also contributed to our understanding of tumor classifications and prompted the evaluation of individualized treatments. However, the rapid development of drug resistance remains a major clinical challenge for the majority of patients with advanced-stage disease, prompting studies that target regenerative subpopulations of resistant cells.

The next few years will see mature data from phase III trials targeting VEGF, including integration with intraperitoneal chemotherapy, as well as numerous phase II trials with diverse molecular-targeted agents. Comparative data among these agents are limited, and selection of high-priority combinations will remain challenging. Future phase III trials will depend on carefully designed randomized phase II studies with criteria for the selection of promising combinations, based on feasibility, tolerability, and efficacy.

References

1. Alberts DS, Green S, Hannigan EV et al (1992) Improved therapeutic index of carboplatin plus cyclophosphamide versus cisplatin plus cyclophosphamide: final report by the Southwest Oncology Group of a phase III randomized trial in stages III and IV ovarian cancer. J Clin Oncol 10:706–717
2. Calvert AH, Newell DR, Gumbrell LA et al (1989) Carboplatin dosage: prospective evaluation of a simple formula based on renal function. J Clin Oncol 7:1748–1756
3. du Bois A, Luck HJ, Meier W et al (2003) Arbeitsgemeinschaft Gynakologische Onkologie Ovarian Cancer Study Group. A randomized clinical trial of cisplatin/paclitaxel versus carboplatin/paclitaxel as first-line treatment of ovarian cancer. J Natl Cancer Inst 95:1320–1329
4. Ozols RF, Bundy BN, Greer BE et al (2003) Phase III trial of carboplatin and paclitaxel compared with cisplatin and paclitaxel in patients with optimally resected stage III ovarian cancer: a Gynecologic Oncology Group study. J Clin Oncol 21:3194–3200
5. Gore M, Mainwaring P, A'Hern R et al (1998) Randomized trial of dose-intensity with single-agent carboplatin in patients with epithelial ovarian cancer. London Gynaecological Oncology Group. J Clin Oncol 16:2426–2434
6. Jakobsen A, Bertelsen K, Andersen JE et al (1997) Dose-effect study of carboplatin in ovarian cancer: a Danish Ovarian Cancer Group study. J Clin Oncol 15:193–198
7. Möbus V, Wandt H, Frickhofen N et al (2007) Phase III trial of high-dose sequential chemotherapy with peripheral blood stem cell support compared with standard dose chemotherapy for first-line treatment of advanced ovarian cancer: intergroup trial of the AGO-Ovar/AIO and EBMT. J Clin Oncol 25:4187–4193

8. McGuire WP, Hoskins WJ, Brady MF et al (1996) Cyclophosphamide and cisplatin compared with paclitaxel and cisplatin in patients with stage III and stage IV ovarian cancer. N Engl J Med 334:1–6

9. Piccart MJ, Bertelsen K, James K et al (2000) Randomized intergroup trial of cisplatin-paclitaxel versus cisplatin-cyclophosphamide in women with advanced epithelial ovarian cancer: three-year results. J Natl Cancer Inst 92:699–708

10. Piccart MJ, Bertelsen K, Stuart G et al (2003) Long-term follow-up confirms a survival advantage of the paclitaxel-cisplatin regimen over the cyclophosphamide-cisplatin combination in advanced ovarian cancer. Int J Gynecol Cancer 13(suppl 2):144–148

11. du Bois A, Quinn M, Thigpen T et al (2005) 2004 consensus statements on the management of ovarian cancer: final document of the 3rd International Gynecologic Cancer Intergroup Ovarian Cancer Consensus Conference (GCIG OCCC 2004). Ann Oncol 16(Suppl 8): viii7–viii12

12. International Collaborative Ovarian Neoplasm Group (2002) Paclitaxel plus carboplatin versus standard chemotherapy with either single-agent carboplatin or cyclophosphamide, doxorubicin, and cisplatin in women with ovarian cancer: the ICON3 randomised trial. Lancet 360:505–515

13. Muggia FM, Braly PS, Brady MF et al (2000) Phase III randomized study of cisplatin versus paclitaxel versus cisplatin and paclitaxel in patients with suboptimal stage III or IV ovarian cancer: a gynecologic oncology group study. J Clin Oncol 18:106–115

14. Parmar MK, Ledermann JA, Colombo N et al (2003) ICON and AGO Collaborators. Paclitaxel plus platinum-based chemotherapy versus conventional platinum-based chemotherapy in women with relapsed ovarian cancer: the ICON4/AGO-OVAR-2.2 trial. Lancet 361: 2099–2106

15. Vasey PA, Jayson GC, Gordon A et al (2004) Phase III randomized trial of docetaxel-carboplatin versus paclitaxel-carboplatin as first-line chemotherapy for ovarian carcinoma. J Natl Cancer Inst 96:1682–1691

16. Fennelly D, Aghajanian C, Shapiro F et al (1997) Phase I and pharmacologic study of paclitaxel administered weekly in patients with relapsed ovarian cancer. J Clin Oncol 15: 187–192

17. Markman M, Blessing J, Rubin SC et al (2006) Phase II trial of weekly paclitaxel (80 mg/m^2) in platinum and paclitaxel-resistant ovarian and primary peritoneal cancers: a Gynecologic Oncology Group study. Gynecol Oncol 101:436–440

18. Katsumata N, Yasuda M, Takahashi F et al (2009) Dose-dense paclitaxel once a week in combination with carboplatin every 3 weeks for advanced ovarian cancer: a phase 3, open-label, randomised controlled trial. Lancet 374:1331–1338

19. du Bois A, Belau A, Wagner U et al (2005) A phase II study of paclitaxel, carboplatin, and gemcitabine in previously untreated patients with epithelial ovarian cancer FIGO stage IC-IV (AGO-OVAR protocol OVAR-8). Gynecol Oncol 96:444–451

20. Look KY, Bookman MA, Schol J et al (2004) Phase I feasibility trial of carboplatin, paclitaxel, and gemcitabine in patients with previously untreated epithelial ovarian or primary peritoneal cancer: a Gynecologic Oncology Group study. Gynecol Oncol 92:93–100

21. Trimble EL, Davis J, DiSaia P et al (2007) Clinical trials in gynecological cancer. Int J Gynecol Cancer 17:547–556

22. Bookman MA, Brady MF, McGuire W et al (2009) Evaluation of new platinum-based treatment regimens in advanced-stage ovarian cancer: a Phase III Trial of the Gynecologic Cancer InterGroup (GCIG). J Clin Oncol 27:1419–1425

23. du Bois A, Weber B, Rochon J et al (2006) Addition of epirubicin as a third drug to carboplatin-paclitaxel in first-line treatment of advanced ovarian cancer: a prospectively randomized gynecologic cancer intergroup trial by the Arbeitsgemeinschaft Gynaekologische Onkologie Ovarian Cancer Study Group and the Groupe d'Investigateurs Nationaux pour l'Etude des Cancers Ovariens. J Clin Oncol 24:1127–1135

24. Hoskins PJ, Vergote I, Stuart G et al (2008) Phase III trial of cisplatin plus topotecan followed by paclitaxel plus carboplatin versus standard carboplatin plus paclitaxel as first-line chemotherapy in women with newly diagnosed advanced epithelial ovarian cancer (EOC) (OV.16). A Gynecologic Cancer Intergroup Study of the NCIC CTG, EORTC GCG, and GEICO. J Clin Oncol 26:Abstract LBA5505

25. Kristensen GB, Vergote I, Stuart G et al (2003) First-line treatment of ovarian cancer FIGO stages IIb-IV with paclitaxel/epirubicin/carboplatin versus paclitaxel/carboplatin. Int J Gynecol Cancer 13(suppl 2):172–177

26. Scarfone G, Scambia G, Raspagliesi F et al (2006) A multicenter, randomized, phase III study comparing paclitaxel/carboplatin (PC) versus topotecan/paclitaxel/carboplatin (TPC) in patients with stage III (residual tumor >1 cm after primary surgery) and IV ovarian cancer (OC). J Clin Oncol 24(suppl 18S):Abstract 5003

27. Bookman MA, McMeekin DS, Fracasso P (2006) Sequence-dependence of hematologic toxicity using carboplatin and topotecan for primary therapy of advanced epithelial ovarian cancer: A phase I study of the Gynecologic Oncology Group. Gynecol Oncol 103: 473–478

28. Guminski AD, Harnett PR, deFazio A (2001) Carboplatin and paclitaxel interact antagonistically in a megakaryoblast cell line – a potential mechanism for paclitaxel-mediated sparing of carboplatin-induced thrombocytopenia. Cancer Chemother Pharmacol 48:229–234

29. Teneriello MG, Tseng PC, Crozier M et al (2009) Phase II evaluation of nanoparticle albumin-bound paclitaxel in platinum-sensitive patients with recurrent ovarian, peritoneal, or fallopian tube cancer. J Clin Oncol 27:1426–1431

30. Dumontet C, Jordan MA, Lee FF (2009) Ixabepilone: targeting beta III-tubulin expression in taxane-resistant malignancies. Mol Cancer Ther 8:17–25

31. Krasner CN, McMeekin DS, Chan S et al (2007) A Phase II study of trabectedin single agent in patients with recurrent ovarian cancer previously treated with platinum-based regimens. Br J Cancer 97:1618–1624

32. Miller DS, Blessing JA, Krasner CN et al (2009) Phase II evaluation of pemetrexed in the treatment of recurrent or persistent platinum-resistant ovarian or primary peritoneal carcinoma: a study of the Gynecologic Oncology Group. J Clin Oncol 27:2686–2691

33. Vergote I, Calvert H, Kania M et al (2009) A randomised, double-blind, phase II study of two doses of pemetrexed in the treatment of platinum-resistant, epithelial ovarian or primary peritoneal cancer. Eur J Cancer 45:1415–1423

34. Hess V, A'Hern R, Nasiri N et al (2004) Mucinous epithelial ovarian cancer: a separate entity requiring specific treatment. J Clin Oncol 22:1040–1044

35. Winter WE 3rd, Maxwell GL, Tian C et al (2007) Prognostic factors for stage III epithelial ovarian cancer: a Gynecologic Oncology Group Study. J Clin Oncol 25:3621–3627

36. Chan JK, Tian C, Monk BJ et al (2008) Prognostic factors for high-risk early-stage epithelial ovarian cancer. A Gynecologic Oncology Group study. Cancer 112:2202–2210

37. Trimbos JB, Parmar M, Vergote I (2003) International Collaborative Ovarian Neoplasm 1 (ICON1) and European Organisation for Research and Treatment of Cancer Collaborators–Adjuvant ChemoTherapy In Ovarian Neoplasm (EORTC–ACTION). International Collaborative Ovarian Neoplasm trial and Adjuvant Chemo Therapy In Ovarian Neoplasm trial: two parallel randomized phase III trials of adjuvant chemotherapy in patients with early-stage ovarian carcinoma. J Natl Cancer Inst 95:105–112

38. Trimbos JB, Vergote I, Bolis G et al (2003) For the EORTC–ACTION collaborators. Impact of adjuvant chemotherapy and surgical staging in early-stage ovarian carcinoma: European Organisation for Research and Treatment of Cancer–Adjuvant ChemoTherapy in Ovarian Neoplasm trial. J Natl Cancer Inst 95:113–125

39. Pohl G, Ho CL, Kurman RJ et al (2005) Inactivation of the mitogen-activated protein kinase pathway as a potential target-based therapy in ovarian serous tumors with KRAS or BRAF mutations. Cancer Res 65:1994–2000

40. Singer G, Stöhr R, Cope L et al (2005) Patterns of p53 mutations separate ovarian serous borderline tumors and low- and high-grade carcinomas and provide support for a new model of ovarian carcinogenesis: a mutational analysis with immunohistochemical correlation. Am J Surg Pathol 29:218–224
41. Ahn NG, Nahreini TS, Tolwinski NS, Resing KA (2001) Pharmacologic inhibitors of MKK1 and MKK2. Meth Enzymol 332:417–431
42. Khokhlatchev AV, Canagarajah B, Wilsbacher J et al (1998) Phosphorylation of the MAP kinase ERK2 promotes its homodimerization and nuclear translocation. Cell 93:605–615
43. Davies BR, Logie A, McKay JS et al (2007) AZD6244 (ARRY-142886), a potent inhibitor of mitogen-activated protein kinase/extracellular signal-regulated kinase kinase ½ kinases: mechanism of action in vivo, pharmacokinetic/pharmacodynamics relationship, and potential for combination in preclinical models. Mol Cancer Ther 6:2209–2219
44. Larue L, Bellacosa A (2005) Epithelial-mesenchymal transition in development and cancer: role of phosphatidylinositol 3' kinase/AKT pathways. Oncogene 24:7443–7454
45. Tothill RW, Tinker AV, George J et al (2008) Novel molecular subtypes of serous and endo-metrioid ovarian cancer linked to clinical outcome. Clin Cancer Res 14:5198–5208
46. Zorn KK, Bonome T, Gangi L et al (2005) Gene expression profiles of serous, endometrioid, and clear cell subtypes of ovarian and endometrial cancer. Clin Cancer Res 11:6422–6430
47. Byrne AT, Ross L, Holash J et al (2003) Vascular endothelial growth factor-trap decreases tumor burden, inhibits ascites, and causes dramatic vascular remodeling in an ovarian cancer model. Clin Cancer Res 9:5721–5728
48. Kumaran GC, Jayson GC, Clamp AR (2009) Antiangiogenic drugs in ovarian cancer. Br J Cancer 100:1–7
49. Martin L, Schilder R (2007) Novel approaches in advancing the treatment of epithelial ovarian cancer: the role of angiogenesis inhibition. J Clin Oncol 25:2894–2901
50. Burger RA, Sill MW, Monk BJ, Greer BE, Sorosky JI (2007) Phase II trial of bevacizumab in persistent or recurrent epithelial ovarian cancer or primary peritoneal cancer: a Gynecologic Oncology Group Study. J Clin Oncol 25:5165–5171
51. Cannistra SA, Matulonis UA, Penson RT et al (2007) Phase II study of bevacizumab in patients with platinum-resistant ovarian cancer or peritoneal serous cancer. J Clin Oncol 25:5180–5186
52. Grothey A, Galanis E (2009) Targeting angiogenesis: progress with anti-VEGF treatment with large molecules. Nat Rev Clin Oncol 6:507–518
53. Martin LP, Hamilton TC, Schilder RJ (2008) Platinum resistance: the role of DNA repair pathways. Clin Cancer Res 14:1291–1295
54. Muggia F (2009) Platinum compounds 30 years after the introduction of cisplatin: implications for the treatment of ovarian cancer. Gynecol Oncol 112:275–281
55. Gore ME, Atkinson RJ, Thomas H et al (2002) A phase II trial of ZD0473 in platinum-pretreated ovarian cancer. Eur J Cancer 38:2416–2420
56. Fracasso PM, Blessing JA, Morgan MA et al (2003) Phase II study of oxaliplatin in platinum-resistant and refractory ovarian cancer: a gynecologic group study. J Clin Oncol 21:2856–2859
57. Glasspool RM, Gore M, Rustin G et al (2009) Randomized phase II study of decitabine in combination with carboplatin compared with carboplatin alone in patients with recurrent advanced ovarian cancer. Clin Oncol 27(suppl; abstr 5562):15s
58. Gossage L, Madhusudan S (2007) Current status of excision repair cross complementing-group 1 (ERCC1) in cancer. Cancer Treat Rev 33:565–577
59. Vilmar A, Sørensen JB (2009) Excision repair cross-complementation group 1 (ERCC1) in platinum-based treatment of non-small cell lung cancer with special emphasis on carboplatin: a review of current literature. Lung Cancer 64:131–139
60. Holzer AK, Howell SB (2006) The internalization and degradation of human copper transporter 1 following cisplatin exposure. Cancer Res 66:10944–10952

61. Glinsky GV (2008) "Stemness" genomics law governs clinical behavior of human cancer: implications for decision making in disease management. J Clin Oncol26:2846–2853
62. Szotek PP, Pieretti-Vanmarcke R, Masiakos PT et al (2006) Ovarian cancer side population defines cells with stem cell-like characteristics and Mullerian Inhibiting Substance responsiveness. Proc Natl Acad Sci USA 103:11154–11159
63. Fojo T, Bates S (2003) Strategies for reversing drug resistance. Oncogene 22:7512–7523
64. Lhommé C, Joly F, Walker JL et al (2008) Phase III study of valspodar (PSC 833) combined with paclitaxel and carboplatin compared with paclitaxel and carboplatin alone in patients with stage IV or suboptimally debulked stage III epithelial ovarian cancer or primary peritoneal cancer. J Clin Oncol 26:2674–2682
65. Sharom FJ (2008) ABC multidrug transporters: structure, function and role in chemoresistance. Pharmacogenomics 9:105–127
66. Bookman MA (2005) Gemcitabine monotherapy in recurrent ovarian cancer: from the bench to the clinic. Int J Gynecol Cancer 15(suppl 1):12–17
67. Galmarini CM, Mackey JR, Dumontet C (2001) Nucleoside analogues: mechanisms of drug resistance and reversal strategies. Leukemia 15:875–890
68. Mini E, Nobili S, Caciagli B et al (2006) Cellular pharmacology of gemcitabine. Ann Oncol 15(suppl 5):v7–v12
69. Bolderson E, Richard DJ, Zhou BB, Khanna KK (2009) Recent advances in cancer therapy targeting proteins involved in DNA double-strand break repair. Clin Cancer Res 15:6314–6320
70. Bryant HE, Schultz N, Thomas HD et al (2005) Specific killing of BRCA2-deficient tumours with inhibitors of poly(ADP-ribose) polymerase. Nature 434:913–917
71. Fong PC, Boss DS, Yap TA et al (2009) Inhibition of poly (ADP-ribose) polymerase in tumors from BRCA mutation carriers. N Engl J Med 361:123–134
72. Esteller M, Silva JM, Dominguez G et al (2000) Promoter hypermethylation and BRCA1 inactivation in sporadic breast and ovarian tumors. J Natl Cancer Inst 92:564–569
73. Hilton JL, Geisler JP, Rathe JA et al (2002) Inactivation of BRCA1 and BRCA2 in ovarian cancer. J Natl Cancer Inst 94:1396–1406
74. Edwards SL, Brough R, Lord CJ (2008) Resistance to therapy caused by intragenic deletion in BRCA2. Nature 451:1111–1115
75. Sakai W, Swisher EM, Karlan BY et al (2008) Secondary mutations as a mechanism of cisplatin resistance in BRCA2-mutated cancers. Nature 451:1116–1120
76. Bolis G, Scarfone G, Polverino G, Raspagliesi F et al (2004) Paclitaxel 175 or 225 mg per meters squared with carboplatin in advanced ovarian cancer: a randomized trial. J Clin Oncol 22:686–690
77. Eisenhauer EA, ten Bokkel Huinink WW, Swenerton KD et al (1994) European-Canadian randomized trial of paclitaxel in relapsed ovarian cancer: high-dose versus low-dose and long versus short infusion. J Clin Oncol 12:2654–2666
78. Omura GA, Brady MF, Look KY et al (2003) Phase III trial of paclitaxel at two dose levels, the higher dose accompanied by filgrastim at two dose levels in platinum-pretreated epithelial ovarian cancer: an intergroup study. J Clin Oncol 21:2843–2848
79. Markman M, Rose PG, Jones E et al (1998) Ninety-six-hour infusional paclitaxel as salvage therapy of ovarian cancer patients previously failing treatment with 3-hour or 24-hour paclitaxel infusion regimens. J Clin Oncol 16:1849–1851
80. Spriggs DR, Brady MF, Vaccarello L et al (2007) Phase III randomized trial of intravenous cisplatin plus a 24- or 96-hour infusion of paclitaxel in epithelial ovarian cancer: a Gynecologic Oncology Group Study. J Clin Oncol 25:4466–4471
81. Alberts DS, Liu PY, Hannigan EV et al (1996) Intraperitoneal cisplatin plus intravenous cyclophosphamide versus intravenous cisplatin plus intravenous cyclophosphamide for stage III ovarian cancer. N Engl J Med 335:1950–1955

82. Armstrong DK, Bundy B, Wenzel L et al (2006) Intraperitoneal cisplatin and paclitaxel in ovarian cancer. N Engl J Med 354:34–43
83. Markman M, Bundy BN, Alberts DS et al (2001) Phase III trial of standard-dose intravenous cisplatin plus paclitaxel versus moderately high-dose carboplatin followed by intravenous paclitaxel and intraperitoneal cisplatin in small-volume stage III ovarian carcinoma: an inter-group study of the Gynecologic Oncology Group, Southwestern Oncology Group, and Eastern Cooperative Oncology Group. J Clin Oncol 19:1001–1007
84. Hess LM, Benham-Hutchins M, Herzog TJ et al (2007) A meta-analysis of the efficacy of intraperitoneal cisplatin for the front-line treatment of ovarian cancer. Int J Gynecol Cancer 17:561–570
85. Jaaback K, Johnson N (2006) Intraperitoneal chemotherapy for the initial management of primary epithelial ovarian cancer. Cochrane Database Syst Rev 25:CD005340
86. Ozols RF, Bookman MA, du Bois A et al (2006) Intraperitoneal cisplatin therapy in ovarian cancer: comparison with standard intravenous carboplatin and paclitaxel. Gynecol Oncol 103:1–6
87. Swart AM, Burdett S, Ledermann J, Mook P, Parmar MK (2008) Why i.p. therapy cannot yet be considered as a standard of care for the first-line treatment of ovarian cancer: a systematic review. Ann Oncol 19:688–695
88. Bolis G, Danese S, Tateo S et al (2006) Epidoxorubicin versus no treatment as consolidation therapy in advanced ovarian cancer: results from a phase II study. Int J Gynecol Cancer 16(suppl 1):74–78
89. De Placido S, Scanbia G, Di Vagno G et al (2004) Topotecan compared with no therapy after response to surgery and carboplatin/paclitaxel in patients with ovarian cancer: Multicenter Italian Trials in Ovarian Cancer (MITO-1) randomized study. J Clin Oncol 22:2635–2642
90. Markman M, Liu PY, Wilczynski S et al (2003) Phase III randomized trial of 12 versus 3 months of maintenance paclitaxel in patients with advanced ovarian cancer after complete response to platinum and paclitaxel-based chemotherapy: a Southwest Oncology Group and Gynecologic Oncology Group trial. J Clin Oncol 21:2460–2465
91. Pfisterer J, Weber B, Reuss A et al (2006) Randomized phase III trial of topotecan following carboplatin and paclitaxel in first-line treatment of advanced ovarian cancer: a gynecologic cancer intergroup trial of the AGO-OVAR and GINECO. J Natl Cancer Inst 98:1036–1045
92. Piccart MJ, Floquet A, Scarfone G et al (2003) Intraperitoneal cisplatin versus no further treatment: 8-year results of EORTC 55875, a randomized phase III study in ovarian cancer patients with a pathologically complete remission after platinum-based intravenous chemotherapy. Int J Gynecol Cancer 13(suppl 2):196–203
93. Alberts DS, Hannigan EV, Liu PY et al (2006) Randomized trial of adjuvant intraperitoneal alpha-interferon in stage III ovarian cancer patients who have no evidence of disease after primary surgery and chemotherapy: an intergroup study. Gynecol Oncol 100:133–138
94. Berek JS, Taylor PT, Gordon A et al (2004) Randomized, placebo-controlled study of orego-vomab for consolidation of clinical remission in patients with advanced ovarian cancer. J Clin Oncol 22:3507–3516
95. Verheijen RH, Massuger LF, Benigno BB et al (2006) Phase III trial of intraperitoneal therapy with yttrium-90-labeled HMFG1 murine monoclonal antibody in patients with epithelial ovarian cancer after a surgically defined complete remission. J Clin Oncol 24:571–578
96. Dowdy SC, Loewen RT, Aletti G, Feitoza SS, Cliby W (2008) Assessment of outcomes and morbidity following diaphragmatic peritonectomy for women with ovarian carcinoma. Gynecol Oncol 109:303–307
97. Eisenkop SM, Spirtos NM, Lin WC (2006) "Optimal" cytoreduction for advanced epithelial ovarian cancer: a commentary. Gynecol Oncol 103:329–335

98. Winter WE 3rd, Maxwell GL, Tian C et al (2008) Tumor residual after surgical cytoreduction in prediction of clinical outcome in stage IV epithelial ovarian cancer: a Gynecologic Oncology Group Study. J Clin Oncol 26:83–89

99. Bristow RE, Eisenhauer EL, Santillan A, Chi DS (2007) Delaying the primary surgical effort for advanced ovarian cancer: a systematic review of neoadjuvant chemotherapy and interval cytoreduction. Gynecol Oncol 104:480–490

100. Rose PG, Nerenstone S, Brady MF et al (2004) Secondary surgical cytoreduction for advanced ovarian carcinoma. N Engl J Med 351:2489–2497

101. van der Burg ME, van Lent M, Buyse M et al (1995) The effect of debulking surgery after induction chemotherapy on the prognosis in advanced epithelial ovarian cancer. Gynecological Cancer Cooperative Group of the European Organization for Research and Treatment of Cancer. N Engl J Med 332:629–634

102. Greer BE, Bundy BN, Ozols RF et al (2005) Implications of second-look laparotomy in the context of optimally resected stage III ovarian cancer: a non-randomized comparison using an explanatory analysis: a Gynecologic Oncology Group study. Gynecol Oncol 99:71–79

103. Curiel TJ, Coukos G, Zou L et al (2004) Specific recruitment of regulatory T cells in ovarian carcinoma fosters immune privilege and predicts reduced survival. Nat Med 10:942–949

104. Zhang L, Conejo-Garcia JR, Katsaros D et al (2003) Intratumoral T cells, recurrence, and survival in epithelial ovarian cancer. N Engl J Med 348:203–213

Principles of Intraperitoneal Chemotherapy

3

Maurie Markman

3.1
Introduction

Despite the completion and publication of the results of three well-designed and conducted phase III randomized trials that revealed the superiority of intraperitoneal, compared to intravenous cisplatin-based chemotherapy employed as primary chemotherapy of small-volume residual advanced ovarian cancer [1–3], there appears to be limited use of this approach outside the setting of clinical trials and major academic medical centers. While a variety of explanations can be offered to this somewhat discouraging state of affairs, it is reasonable to speculate that many clinicians do not fully appreciate the underlying rationale and basic principles supporting this method of drug delivery in the management of ovarian cancer. Such considerations actually provide strong support for the validity of the outcomes observed in the completed randomized trials.

In this chapter, the principles of intraperitoneal drug delivery will be presented, highlighting both the potential benefits and limitations of this strategy in the management of ovarian cancer.

3.2
Rationale for the Delivery of Antineoplastic Agents by the Intraperitoneal Route as a Treatment for Intraperitoneal Malignancies

3.2.1
Anatomic Location of the Cancer

It was recognized in the earliest years of the development of antineoplastic agents that it was reasonable to consider the direct delivery of these drugs into the abdominal cavity in the management of cancers known to involve this body compartment [4, 5]. Unfortunately,

M. Markman
Department of Gynecologic Medical Oncology, The University of Texas M.D.
Anderson Cancer Center, 1515 Holcombe Boulevard, Houston, TX 77030, USA
e-mail: mmarkman@mdanderson.org

D.S. Alberts et al. (eds.), *Intraperitoneal Therapy for Ovarian Cancer*,
DOI: 10.1007/978-3-642-12130-2_3, © Springer-Verlag Berlin Heidelberg 2010

the drugs available in the 1960s (e.g., cytotoxic alkylating agents) had limited activity against malignancies that were principally confined to the peritoneal cavity (including ovarian cancer). Further, at least some of these drugs were clearly locally toxic (e.g., recognized vesicant or irritant properties). In addition, any benefit observed in the control of malignant ascites in the initial reports of this strategy may have actually resulted from a sclerosing effect, rather than from a direct biological impact of the agent on the malignant cell population.

However, despite this initial experience, it remained a valid hypothesis that the instillation of an antineoplastic drug into the peritoneal cavity has the potential to produce clinically relevant cytotoxicity secondary to the uptake of the agent into the malignant cell population by free-surface diffusion from the body compartment. Other factors (discussed below) were later found to substantially influence both the drugs and clinical settings, where this approach can be realistically considered a viable therapeutic option in disease management.

3.2.2
General Physiology of the Peritoneal Cavity Relevant for Intraperitoneal Antineoplastic Drug Delivery

Considerable preclinical efforts have been devoted to defining the features that characterize the relationship between drugs and the peritoneal cavity following instillation of an agent directly into that body compartment [6–9]. Much of the early basic research in this area was directed toward understanding the normal physiology of the peritoneal cavity as the principles of, and technology associated with, peritoneal dialysis in the management of kidney failure were being developed.

In general, it is appropriate to conclude that water soluble agents instilled into the peritoneal cavity will exit the compartment slower than lipid soluble agents. It is also the case that the greater the molecular weight of an agent, the longer will it remain within the peritoneal cavity. Of considerable conceptual relevance, the longer an agent persists in a biologically active form within the peritoneal cavity, the greater the antineoplastic effects, and the more rapidly it is cleared from systemic circulation, the more reduced is the systemic exposure to the agent.

Similarly, and of particular importance to both the efficacy and toxicity of intraperitoneal chemotherapy, antineoplastic agents that are rapidly and extensively metabolized to nontoxic and biologically inactive metabolites during their initial passage through the liver are predicted to demonstrate the greatest pharmacokinetic advantage for peritoneal cavity exposures compared to the concentrations observed within the systemic compartment [7]. Conversely, agents that are not metabolized, or undergo minimal changes in the liver, are predicted to show a far more modest difference in the overall measured exposure of the body compartment compared to those observed within the systemic circulation [7]. It has long been recognized that drug uptake from the peritoneal cavity is principally via the portal circulation [8, 9]. Thus, following intraperitoneal administration, these agents will pass directly through the liver prior to their entry into the systemic compartment (e.g., systemic circulation).

3.2.3
Evidence of Concentration-Dependent Biological Activity of an Antineoplastic Agent

It is reasonable to suggest that the major theoretical advantage associated with intraperitoneal antineoplastic drug delivery is the opportunity to expose tumor cells present within the abdominal cavity to modestly or even substantially higher concentrations of an active anticancer agent (increase in the peak level), and for such exposure to potentially persist for considerably longer periods of time (increase in the total AUC [area-under-the-concentration-vs.-time curve]) than safely possible following systemic administration [10]. Therefore, antineoplastic agents that demonstrate significantly enhanced biologic activity in preclinical models at levels (peak or total AUC) that are not achievable following systemic delivery, due to the production of excessive toxicity (e.g., bone marrow suppression, neuropathy, nephrotoxicity) , are ideal drugs to be examined for a potential role of intraperitoneal delivery.

For example, preclinical evaluation has revealed that when some ovarian cancer cells become resistant to cisplatin, the actual degree of resistance is really quite modest (2- to 4-fold) compared to the "sensitive" tumor cell population [11]. Unfortunately, it is not realistically possible to routinely administer either cisplatin or carboplatin systemically at doses or concentrations that even "double" that which is employed in clinical practice due to the production of unquestionably unacceptable side effects [12, 13].

However, formal evaluation of both cisplatin and carboplatin delivered by the intraperitoneal route has revealed a pharmacokinetic advantage of approximately 10- to 20-fold in the peritoneal cavity as compared to systemic exposure [14–19]. As a result, it is possible that a clinically relevant degree of "platinum resistance" can be overcome within the peritoneal cavity because of the concentrations attained in the peritoneal cavity following regional administration which are not achievable with the delivery of the drug to the tumor by systemic administration. It is important to emphasize that what has been presented here was originally a hypothesis for the potential superiority of intraperitoneal platinum instillation in the treatment of ovarian cancer, that was subsequently tested in randomized phase III clinical trials [1–3].

An additional theoretical benefit of intraperitoneal drug delivery can be advanced for agents, such as paclitaxel, which are extensively metabolized during their first passage through the liver (in contrast to the platinum agents which undergo minimal or no change in the liver) [20]. Not only are substantial differences between peak levels and total AUC exposures between the peritoneal cavity and systemic compartments observed (greater than 1,000-fold) [21, 22], but cytotoxic drug concentrations of taxanes may persist within the intraperitoneal space for prolonged periods of time [21].

For example, in a phase I clinical trial of paclitaxel administered by the intraperitoneal route on a weekly schedule, investigators measured the concentration of the agent present within the peritoneal cavity 5–7 days after the last treatment cycle. Peritoneal cavity levels were found to be several times greater than the peak concentrations within the systemic compartment achieved when paclitaxel is delivered by the intravenous route [21]. These data suggest that following a single dose of intraperitoneal paclitaxel, the cavity is exposed to highly cytotoxic concentrations of this cycle-specific antineoplastic agent for prolonged periods, an outcome that would not be possible with systemic delivery due to the production of excessive bone marrow suppression. Again, whether or not this provocative biological effect can be translated into clinical benefit for patients treated with paclitaxel delivered by the intraperitoneal route is a hypothesis, which was later tested in a phase III randomized trial [2].

3.3
Limitations of Intraperitoneal Antineoplastic Drug Delivery

3.3.1
Local Toxicity of Antineoplastic Agents

The experience with the intraperitoneal administration of cytotoxic alkylating agents emphasizes the importance of documenting the local side effects of any agent being considered for regional therapy. In fact, while a strong preclinical and clinical rationale may be presented for a particular agent for intraperitoneal delivery, toxicities unique to this route of delivery may simply prevent its use in this manner [23]. For example, both doxorubicin and mitoxantrone have been shown to be more active in preclinical model systems at concentrations achievable following intraperitoneal, but not systemic, administration [10, 24]. Unfortunately, these agents produced excessive local toxicity (e.g., pain, adhesion formation, bowel obstruction) when delivered intraperitoneally, which prevents their use in routine clinical practice [25, 26]. These experiences clearly demonstrate that the safety of any single-agent or combination regional chemotherapy regimen must be documented prior to embarking on clinical trials examining the efficacy of the regimen.

3.3.2
Adequacy of Drug Distribution

In contrast to systemic drug administration, where it can be reasonably accepted that the drug will reach the tumor by capillary flow (even if it is completely unknown if the delivered concentration will be adequate to produce a desired biological effect), it would not be rational to simply assume that drug instilled into the peritoneal cavity will disperse to all areas of this body compartment [27]. In fact, the presence of adhesions, resulting from surgical trauma, the cancer, or a subsequent local inflammatory effect of the antineoplastic agent itself, may interfere with the distribution of the instilled drug-containing fluid volume.

Despite these concerns, the results of numerous clinical trials have provided convincing evidence that as long as it is possible to safely administer treatment in a volume of approximately one to two liters, then there does not appear to be a pattern of disease recurrence or progression within the cavity. Conversely, if it is not possible to infuse this volume due to patients' complaints of pain or extremely slow entry of the treatment-containing fluid, then it is reasonable to assume in this setting that intraperitoneal therapy should not be continued. Unfortunately, the development of this clinical scenario generally signifies the presence of significant intraperitoneal adhesions, which will limit the efficacy of regional delivery.

3.3.3
Limited Direct Penetration of Antineoplastic Agents into Tumor Masses

Perhaps, the major factor defining the clinical settings where intraperitoneal drug delivery is a rational management strategy for patients with ovarian cancer is the demonstrated limited penetration of antineoplastic agents directly into solid neoplastic or normal tissues. This critically important issue has been examined employing a number of drugs, including 5-fluorouracil, methotrexate, vincristine, doxorubicin, cisplatin, and carboplatin [24, 28–31].

While the results of these studies have varied, it is appropriate to conclude that direct antineoplastic drug penetration into solid tissue by free-surface diffusion is limited to a distance of several cell layers to a maximum of a few millimeters from the cell surface. As a result, it is reasonable to conclude that patients with microscopic disease only or those with very small-volume residual macroscopic ovarian cancers (e.g., less than 0.5–1 cm in maximum tumor diameter) would be most likely to have clinical benefit from regional drug delivery.

However, it is also important to acknowledge that following initial successful reduction in the size of mass lesions following delivery of drug to tumor by capillary flow, previous "large" ovarian tumor masses may be substantially reduced in volume such that the remaining "smaller-sized" malignant cell populations may be far more susceptible to the impact of the increased local concentrations present during subsequent intraperitoneal drug delivery. For example, a particular ovarian cancer patient may have several 2–3 cm (maximal diameter) residual tumor masses remaining within the peritoneal cavity following an attempt at initial surgical cytoreduction (suboptimal residual disease). Considering the recognized fact that 70–80% of patients with ovarian cancer achieve major objective responses to platinum-based chemotherapy [32], if this woman begins cytotoxic therapy with a regimen that includes intraperitoneal cisplatin, it is reasonable to hypothesize that following one or several cycles of such therapy, the volume of any remaining tumor masses will be substantially smaller than when the treatment program was initiated. At this point, the high local platinum concentrations bathing the cavity may favorably impact the overall effectiveness of the therapeutic regimen [33]. As a result, the decision to limit intraperitoneal administration in ovarian cancer only to women with small-volume residual disease following surgical cytoreduction may not be justified in all clinical settings. In fact, existing clinical data provide provocative support for this hypothesis [1, 33].

3.3.4
Importance of Drug Delivery by Capillary Flow

One of the most important questions, and concerns, associated with intraperitoneal antineoplastic drug delivery is that of the impact of this strategy on the concentration of a particular agent reaching the cancer via capillary flow following regional administration. In fact, it is reasonable to suggest that if the use of this route of delivery reduces the extent of exposure of the tumor to a particular agent through capillary flow, then employing this strategy may conceivably negatively impact the overall outcome of a treatment program. However, as previously noted, for the platinum agents (cisplatin and carboplatin), it has been demonstrated that the concentration of biologically active drug reaching systemic circulation following intraperitoneal delivery is essentially equivalent to that achieved if the same dose and concentration had been administered by the intravenous route [14–19]. Therefore, it is reasonable to conclude that there should be no realistic concern that treating an ovarian cancer patient with either cisplatin or carboplatin by the intraperitoneal route will result in a reduction in the concentration of the agents reaching the malignancy by capillary flow.

This conclusion would not necessarily be justified for paclitaxel. Existing data have provided conflicting results regarding the concentration of the active drug present within the systemic compartment following intraperitoneal therapy. Older studies noted quite limited systemic concentrations of paclitaxel with regional delivery [21, 22], perhaps explaining the quite modest degree of bone marrow suppression observed with this treatment strategy [34]. However, more recent data have suggested that it may be possible to achieve clinically relevant cytotoxic concentrations of paclitaxel within the systemic circulation after intraperitoneal administration [35]. Additional research is needed to confirm this provocative observation.

For any new agent considered for exclusively intraperitoneal administration, it will be important to determine whether it is possible to achieve adequate concentrations of the drug within the systemic compartment following regional delivery. If the answer is no, and the goal of the particular treatment program is to maximize the total exposure of tumor to the agent, then both systemic and intraperitoneal administration should be employed.

3.3.5
Other Relevant Issues Defining the Use of Intraperitoneal Chemotherapy

Additional concerns regarding the delivery of intraperitoneal therapy as a management strategy for women with ovarian cancer include the time and effort required for the successful implementation of this approach as compared to standard intravenous treatment and unique questions related to the special requirements for peritoneal cavity access [36]. Critically important surgical issues related to the appropriate timing of initiating regional drug delivery and the way in which intraperitoneal drug delivery devices are optimally placed will be discussed in subsequent chapters in this book.

3.4
Conclusion

The intraperitoneal administration of antineoplastic agents for the treatment of ovarian cancer is based on sound pharmacokinetic principles [7], knowledge of the natural history of ovarian cancer [37, 38], and an understanding of the anatomy and physiology of this body cavity. However, it is also important to acknowledge that there are critically relevant clinical and biological factors that both define and realistically limit those settings where regional drug delivery is a rational approach in the management of this malignancy.

References

1. Alberts DS, Liu PY, Hannigan EV, O'Toole R, Williams SD, Young JA, Franklin EW, Clarke-Pearson DL, Malviya VK, DuBeshter B (1996) Intraperitoneal cisplatin plus intravenous cyclophosphamide versus intravenous cisplatin plus intravenous cyclophosphamide for stage III ovarian cancer. N Engl J Med 335:1950–1955
2. Armstrong DK, Bundy B, Wenzel L, Huang HQ, Baergen R, Lele S, Copeland LJ, Walker JL, Burger RA (2006) Intraperitoneal cisplatin and paclitaxel in ovarian cancer. N Engl J Med 354:34–43
3. Markman M, Bundy BN, Alberts DS, Fowler JM, Clark-Pearson DL, Carson LF, Wadler S, Sickel J (2001) Phase III trial of standard-dose intravenous cisplatin plus paclitaxel versus moderately high-dose carboplatin followed by intravenous paclitaxel and intraperitoneal cisplatin in small-volume stage III ovarian carcinoma: an intergroup study of the Gynecologic Oncology Group, Southwestern Oncology Group, and Eastern Cooperative Oncology Group. J Clin Oncol 19:1001–1007
4. Suhrland LG, Weisberger AS (1965) Intracavitary 5-fluorouracil in malignant effusions. Arch Intern Med 116:431–433
5. Weisberger AS, Levine B, Storaasli JP (1955) Use of nitrogen mustard in treatment of serous effusions of neoplastic origin. JAMA 159:1704–1707
6. Dedrick RL (1985) Theoretical and experimental bases of intraperitoneal chemotherapy. Semin Oncol 12:1–6
7. Dedrick RL, Myers CE, Bungay PM, DeVita VT Jr (1978) Pharmacokinetic rationale for peritoneal drug administration in the treatment of ovarian cancer. Cancer Treat Rep 62:1–11
8. Kraft AR, Tompkins RK, Jesseph JE (1968) Peritoneal electrolyte absorption: analysis of portal, systemic venous and lymphatic transport. Surgery 64:148–153
9. Lukas G, Brindle SD, Greengard P (1971) The route of absorption of intraperitoneally administered compounds. J Pharmacol Exp Ther 178:562–564
10. Alberts DS, Young L, Mason N, Salmon SE (1985) In vitro evaluation of anticancer drugs against ovarian cancer at concentrations achievable by intraperitoneal administration. Semin Oncol 12:38–42
11. Andrews PA, Velury S, Mann SC, Howell SB (1988) cis-Diamminedichloroplatinum(II) accumulation in sensitive and resistant human ovarian carcinoma cells. Cancer Res 48:68–73
12. Gore M, Mainwaring P, A'Hern R, MacFarlane V, Slevin M, Harper P, Osborne R, Mansi J, Blake P, Wiltshaw E, Shepherd J (1998) Randomized trial of dose-intensity with single-agent carboplatin in patients with epithelial ovarian cancer. London Gynaecological Oncology Group. J Clin Oncol 16:2426–2434
13. McGuire WP, Hoskins WJ, Brady MF, Homesley HD, Creasman WT, Berman ML, Ball H, Berek JS, Woodward J (1995) Assessment of dose-intensive therapy in suboptimally debulked ovarian cancer: a Gynecologic Oncology Group study. J Clin Oncol 13:1589–1599
14. Casper ES, Kelsen DP, Alcock NW, Lewis JL Jr (1983) Ip cisplatin in patients with malignant ascites: pharmacokinetic evaluation and comparison with the IV route. Cancer Treat Rep 67:235–238
15. Degregorio MW, Lum BL, Holleran WM, Wilbur BJ, Sikic BI (1986) Preliminary observations of intraperitoneal carboplatin pharmacokinetics during a phase I study of the Northern California Oncology Group. Cancer Chemother Pharmacol 18:235–238
16. Elferink F, van der Vijgh WJ, Klein I, ten Bokkel Huinink WW, Dubbelman R, McVie JG (1988) Pharmacokinetics of carboplatin after intraperitoneal administration. Cancer Chemother Pharmacol 21:57–60
17. Howell SB, Pfeifle CL, Wung WE, Olshen RA, Lucas WE, Yon JL, Green M (1982) Intraperitoneal cisplatin with systemic thiosulfate protection. Ann Intern Med 97:845–851

18. Lopez JA, Krikorian JG, Reich SD, Smyth RD, Lee FH, Issell BF (1985) Clinical pharmacology of intraperitoneal cisplatin. Gynecol Oncol 20:1–9
19. Pretorius RG, Hacker NF, Berek JS, Ford LC, Hoeschele JD, Butler TA, Lagasse LD (1983) Pharmacokinetics of Ip cisplatin in refractory ovarian carcinoma. Cancer Treat Rep 67: 1085–1092
20. Rowinsky EK, Donehower RC (1995) Paclitaxel (taxol). N Engl J Med 332:1004–1014
21. Francis P, Rowinsky E, Schneider J, Hakes T, Hoskins W, Markman M (1995) Phase I feasibility and pharmacologic study of weekly intraperitoneal paclitaxel: a Gynecologic Oncology Group Pilot study. J Clin Oncol 13:2961–2967
22. Markman M, Rowinsky E, Hakes T, Reichman B, Jones W, Lewis JL Jr, Rubin S, Curtin J, Barakat R, Phillips M et al (1992) Phase I trial of intraperitoneal taxol: a Gynecologic Oncology Group study. J Clin Oncol 10:1485–1491
23. Litterst CL, Collins JM, Lowe MC, Arnold ST, Powell DM, Guarino AM (1982) Local and systemic toxicity resulting from large-volume Ip administration of doxorubicin in the rat. Cancer Treat Rep 66:157–161
24. Ozols RF, Locker GY, Doroshow JH, Grotzinger KR, Myers CE, Young RC (1979) Pharmacokinetics of adriamycin and tissue penetration in murine ovarian cancer. Cancer Res 39:3209–3214
25. Markman M, George M, Hakes T, Reichman B, Hoskins W, Rubin S, Jones W, Almadrones L, Lewis JL Jr (1990) Phase II trial of intraperitoneal mitoxantrone in the management of refractory ovarian cancer. J Clin Oncol 8:146–150
26. Roboz J, Jacobs AJ, Holland JF, Deppe G, Cohen CJ (1981) Intraperitoneal infusion of doxorubicin in the treatment of gynecologic carcinomas. Med Pediatr Oncol 9:245–250
27. Litterst CL, Torres IJ, Arnold S, McGunagle D, Furner R, Sikic BI, Guarino AM (1982) Absorption of antineoplastic drugs following large-volume Ip administration of rats. Cancer Treat Rep 66:147–155
28. Durand RE (1981) Flow cytometry studies of intracellular adriamycin in multicell spheroids in vitro. Cancer Res 41:3495–3498
29. Los G, Mutsaers PH, van der Vijgh WJ, Baldew GS, de Graaf PW, McVie JG (1989) Direct diffusion of cis-diamminedichloroplatinum(II) in intraperitoneal rat tumors after intraperitoneal chemotherapy: a comparison with systemic chemotherapy. Cancer Res 49:3380–3384
30. Los G, Verdegaal EM, Mutsaers PH, McVie JG (1991) Penetration of carboplatin and cisplatin into rat peritoneal tumor nodules after intraperitoneal chemotherapy. Cancer Chemother Pharmacol 28:159–165
31. West GW, Weichselbau R, Little JB (1980) Limited penetration of methotrexate into human osteosarcoma spheroids as a proposed model for solid tumor resistance to adjuvant chemotherapy. Cancer Res 40:3665–3668
32. Covens A, Carey M, Bryson P, Verma S, Fung Kee FM, Johnston M (2002) Systematic review of first-line chemotherapy for newly diagnosed postoperative patients with stage II, III, or IV epithelial ovarian cancer. Gynecol Oncol 85:71–80
33. Markman M (2008) Critical thinking: an essential role in both the conduct and interpretation of gynecologic cancer clinical research. Gynecol Oncol 108:462–465
34. Markman M, Brady MF, Spirtos NM, Hanjani P, Rubin SC (1998) A phase II trial of intraperitoneal paclitaxel in carcinoma of the ovary, tube and peritoneum: a Gynecologic Oncology Group study. J Clin Oncol 16:2620–2624
35. Krasner CN, Seiden MV, Fuller AF, Roche M, Verrill CL, D'Amato F, Tretyakov O, Tyburski K, Matulonis UA, Supko JG (2006) Pharmacokinetic analysis of an all intraperitoneal carboplatin and paclitaxel regimen in ovarian cancer patients demonstrates favorable systemic bioavailability of both agents. J Clin Oncol 24(18S):257
36. Walker JL, Armstrong D, Huang HQ, Fowler J, Webster K, Burger R, Clarke-Pearson D (2006) Intraperitoneal catheter outcomes in a phase III trial of intravenous versus intraperitoneal

chemotherapy in optimal stage III ovarian and primary peritoneal cancer: a Gynecologic Oncology Group study. Gynecol Oncol 100:27–32

37. Bergman F (1966) Carcinoma of the ovary: a clinicopathological study of 86 autopsied cases with special reference to mode of spread. Acta Obstet Gynecol Scand 45:211–231

38. Dauplat J, Hacker NF, Nieberg RK, Berek JS, Rose TP, Sagae S (1987) Distant metastases in epithelial ovarian carcinoma. Cancer 60:1561–1566

Intraperitoneal Chemotherapy: Phase III Trials

4

David S. Alberts and Mary C. Clouser

4.1
Introduction

It is well documented that epithelial-type ovarian cancer growth remains within the intraperitoneal (IP) space for the majority of its natural history, making even advanced disease (e.g., stage III) amenable to regional therapy. The concept of IP delivery of chemotherapy goes back more than 40 years to the bioengineer, Robert Dedrick, whose research group at the National Institutes of Health developed animal and mathematical models to describe the disposition of cytotoxic agents administered directly into the IP space [1]. Most notably, his preclinical research led to the "belly bath" as a way of delivering cell-cycle specific agents by continuous 4 h infusions, leading to phase I/II clinical trials of IP 5-fluorouracil and methotrexate in patients with advanced ovarian cancer at the National Cancer Institute (NCI) [2, 3].

Knowledge of Dr. Dedrick's research at the National Institutes of Health and Dr. Speyer's and Dr. Myer's clinical phase I/II research at the NCI led to the research by Dr. Howell and Dr. Markman at the University of California-San Diego and Dr. Casper and colleagues at Memorial Sloan Kettering Cancer Center and Cornell University Medical College [4–6]. They performed a series of groundbreaking pharmacokinetic and phase I/II IP clinical trials, testing various doses and dosing schedules for the promising, but extremely toxic, intraperitoneally administered drug, cisplatin. These studies established the safety, pharmacokinetics, and potential efficacy of an IP cisplatin dose of 100 mg/m^2 administered in 2 L of saline every 3 weeks to patients with stage III, optimally resected ovarian cancer. Furthermore, Dr. Markman, through work completed at Memorial Sloan Kettering, and Dr. Francis, in the Gynecologic Oncology group (GOG), performed phase II and phase I studies, respectively, of IP paclitaxel that documented the safety and efficacy of low, weekly 60 mg/m^2 doses of this agent in patients with persistent, surgically resected ovarian cancer (at second-look surgery) [7, 8]. As with IP cisplatin, the paclitaxel doses were administered in 2 L of 0.9% saline over 1 h with no attempt at IP fluid removal.

D.S. Alberts (✉) and M.C. Clouser
Director, Arizona Cancer Center, University of Arizona,
Tucson, AZ 85724-5024, USA
e-mail: dalberts@azcc.arizona.edu; mclouser@email.arizona.edu

D.S. Alberts et al. (eds.), *Intraperitoneal Therapy for Ovarian Cancer*,
DOI: 10.1007/978-3-642-12130-2_4, © Springer-Verlag Berlin Heidelberg 2010

The research efforts to establish the validity of IP therapy continued through the 1980s and the early 1990s in the form of phase I and limited, uncontrolled phase II clinical trials of intraperitoneally administered single agents (including cisplatin, paclitaxel, fluorodeoxyridine, and multiple other agents active intravenously in recurrent ovarian cancer) [6–9]. Given the proper, conservative approach to drug development for ovarian cancer, these single arm phase II trials seemed to go on endlessly until Dr. Alberts and colleagues submitted a phase III trial protocol proposal in the Southwest Oncology Group (SWOG) for National Cancer Institute-Division of Cancer Treatment-Cancer Therapy Evaluation Program (NCI-DCT-CTEP) review in 1984. At the American Society of Clinical Oncology meeting in May 1985, the CTEP leadership called a meeting of the SWOG, Eastern Cooperative Oncology Group (ECOG), and GOG leadership to launch this pivotal phase III intergroup trial of IP cisplatin/intravenous (IV) cyclophosphamide vs. IV cisplatin/IV cyclophosphamide. This trial required considerable financial support, which was facilitated by Dr. Canetta and Dr. Clark on behalf of Bristol-Myers Squibb and Dr. Coltman, Jr., Chair of the SWOG. Unfortunately, this phase III trial was not a U.S. Food and Drug Administration (FDA) registration trial for IP cisplatin. If it had been, its "pure" design (i.e., equal doses of IP and IV administered drugs with identical IV administered drugs and doses) might have moved the entire regional therapy field ahead more rapidly and secured Medicare reimbursement for IP drug administration at an earlier date.

4.2
SWOG 8501/GOG 0104/EST 3885

SWOG 8501, GOG 0104, EST 3885 began recruitment in 1986 and required a national educational effort to train gynecologic, medical, and nurse oncologists concerning the proper placement and selection of peritoneal catheters, administration of both IV and IP fluids to assure patient safety, and the use of modern supportive care modalities for enhanced patient tolerance.

This intergroup phase III trial was designed as shown in Fig. 4.1. Patient eligibility included: (1) FIGO stage III epithelial-type ovarian cancer; (2) total abdominal

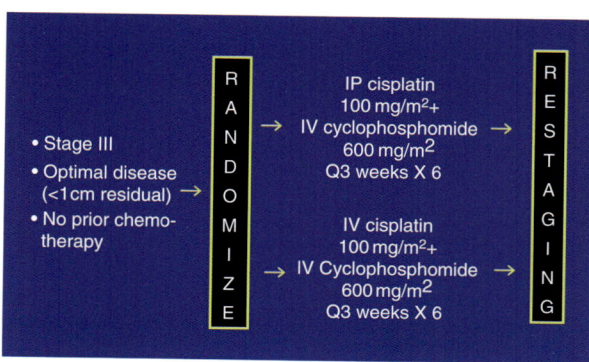

Fig. 4.1 IP cisplatin plus IV cyclophosphamide vs. IV cisplatin plus IV cyclophosphamide for stage III ovarian cancer (SWOG 8501/GOG 0104/EST 3885) [10]

hysterectomy, bilateral salpingo-oophorectomy, partial omentectomy, and resection of all IP tumor masses down to <1 cm; (3) performance status 0–2 (SWOG). After surgery, 654 patients were randomized to either IV or IP cisplatin (100 mg/m^2), plus IV cyclophosphamide (600 mg/m^2) every 3 weeks for six cycles [10]. Of these, 546 were eligible for study. The estimated median survival was significantly longer ($p = 0.02$) in the group receiving IP cisplatin (49 months; 95% confidence interval (CI), 42–56 months) than in the group receiving IV cisplatin (41 months; 95% CI, 34–47 months). The risk of death was lower in the IP group than the IV group (hazard ratio, 0.76; 95% CI, 0.61–0.96; $p = 0.02$). A total of 297 patients with no clinical evidence of disease at the end of chemotherapy underwent adequate second-look surgery. The rate of complete pathological responses was 36% in the IV group and 47% in the IP group. Of extreme interest, as shown in Table 4.1, the IP patient group experienced significantly less granulocytopenia ($p = 0.002$), tinnitus ($p = 0.01$), hearing loss ($p < 0.001$), and neuromuscular effects at the end of treatment ($p = 0.02$). Thus, contrary to conventional wisdom, IP cisplatin is significantly less toxic than IV cisplatin, when administered in equivalent doses. This is not surprising in that cisplatin's hematologic and neurologic toxicity potential, like most cytotoxic drugs, is highly correlated with its postadministration peak serum concentration. It is well documented that IP cisplatin (and all other IP drugs used in the management of ovarian cancer)

Table 4.1 Frequency of adverse events (grade ≥3) during any course of treatment in SWOG 8501

Toxicity	Intravenous group ($n = 276$) %	Intraperitoneal group ($n = 250$) %	p-Value
Anemia (<8.0 g of hemoglobin/dL)	25	26	0.84
Granulocytopenia (<1,000 granulocytes/mm^2)	69	56	0.002
Leukopenia (>2,000 white cells/mm^2)	50	40	0.04
Thrombocytopenia (<50,000 platelets/mm^2)	9	8	0.64
Abdominal pain	2	18	<0.001
Fever	5	6	0.45
Tinnitus	14	7	0.01
Hearing loss	15	5	<0.001
Neuromuscular effects	21	16	0.18
Neuromuscular effects at the end of treatment[a]	25	15	0.02
Pulmonary effects	0.4	3	0.002

Adapted from Alberts et al. [10]

[a]A total of 201 patients in the intravenous group and 175 in the intraperitoneal group completed five or six courses of treatment (no significant differences between groups)

is associated with extremely low peak serum concentrations as compared to those achieved with identical IV cisplatin doses [4, 5].

Although not previously published, the rate of pathological complete remission in the SWOG 8501/GOG 0104/EST 3885 patients who had microscopic-only residual disease after primary cytoreductive surgery was 80% vs. 56% in those patients treated with IP vs. IV cisplatin (and who were found to have microscopic-only disease after primary surgery). Investigators critical of SWOG 8501 final results have claimed that there were errors in the efficacy data, because there was no significant improvement in survival in the IP cisplatin subset who had microscopic residual disease. However, the women who had microscopic-only residual disease after primary cytoreduction surgery clearly had prolonged survival compared to those with macroscopic residual disease, supporting the validity of the surgical staging procedures in SWOG 8501/GOG 0105/EST 3885.

Another criticism of the results of SWOG-8501/GOG-0104/EST-3885 relates to the absence of paclitaxel in both the IP and IV drug combinations. Cyclophosphamide has long been removed as an appropriate first-line therapy drug for advanced ovarian cancer; nevertheless, the major lesson learned from SWOG 8501/GOG 0104/EST 3885 is that regional administration vs. IV administration of an active agent (i.e., cisplatin) is associated with significantly increased survival and decreased systemic toxicity.

4.3
GOG 0114/SWOG 9227/ECOG-GO 114

The success of SWOG 8501/GOG 0104/EST 3885 led directly to the design by the GOG, in concert with the SWOG and the ECOG, of a follow-up phase III trial to test combinations of IV paclitaxel plus either IV cisplatin or IP cisplatin. In the meantime, IV carboplatin had proven as effective as and less toxic than IV cisplatin in the management of patients with advanced ovarian cancer, and as a result, figured into the design of GOG 0114/SWOG 9227/ECOG-GO 114 [11]. As shown in Fig. 4.2, the control arm of this trial, as required by NCI-DCT-CTEP, was the combination of IV cisplatin plus IV

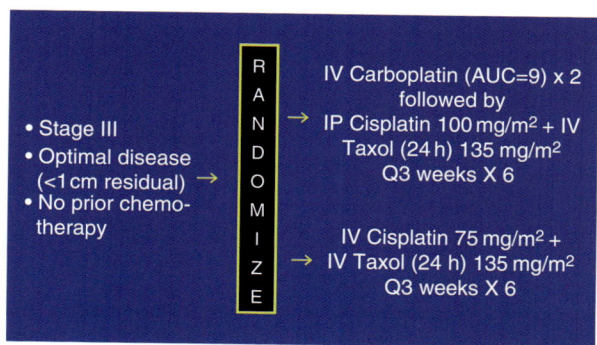

Fig. 4.2 Phase III trial of standard-dose IV cisplatin plus paclitaxel vs. moderately high-dose carboplatin followed by IV paclitaxel and IP cisplatin in small-volume stage III ovarian carcinoma (GOG 0114/SWOG 9227/ECOG-GO 114) [13]

paclitaxel, in that the results of GOG 0158 (i.e., IV cisplatin/IV paclitaxel vs. IV carbo-platin/IV paclitaxel) had not yet been published [12]. The experimental arm of this trial consisted of two IV cycles of moderately high-dose carboplatin (AUC=9 mg min/mL), given initially to reduce IP tumor masses to less than 1 cm individual plaques prior to starting IP cisplatin. The initial two carboplatin doses were to be followed by six cycles of IP cisplatin (100 mg/m^2) on day 1 plus IV paclitaxel 135 mg/m^2 (over 24 h) on day 2 of each 21-day cycle for six cycles. Eligibility for this study was virtually identical to that of SWOG 8501/GOG 0104/EST 3885.

Five hundred and twenty three patients were randomized to the two treatment arms of GOG 0114/SWOG 9227/ECOG-GO 114, of which 462 patients were assessable [13]. At the time of the analysis, 24.7% of those randomized to the control arm had no evidence of disease, compared to 31.9% on the experimental IP arm (Table 4.2). The median progres-sion-free survival for patients in the experimental IP/IV arm was 27.9 months compared with 22.2 months in the standard IV arm (relative risk 0.78, log rank $p=0.01$, one tailed). These progression-free survival data correlated well with the overall survival data [13]. At the time of the analysis, 45.4% of patients on the standard IV arm were alive compared with 53.6% randomized to the IP/IV arm. The median survival duration on the standard IV arm was 52.2 months, compared with 63.2 months on the experimental IP/IV arm (log rank, $p=0.05$, one tailed). The death hazard ratio for the IP to IV treatment groups was 0.81 (90% CI, 0.65–1.00, $p=0.05$).

Of note, 6.8% of the patients randomized to the experimental IP/IV arm did not receive any IP therapy, whereas an additional 18.3% of these patients received only two cycles or less of IP administration, mainly because of increased myelotoxicity experienced during the initial two cycles of IV carboplatin. Table 4.3 shows the toxicities observed on the two study arms. There was significantly more grade 4 neutropenia in the experimental IP/IV arm.

Table 4.2 Survival outcomes of GOG 0114/SWOG 9227/ECOG-GO 114

	IV cisplatin/IV paclitaxel	Carboplatin/IP cisplatin/IV paclitaxel	p-Value
Progression-free survival			
Percent	24.7	31.9	
Months	22.2	27.9	0.01
Hazard ratio (adjusted) for recurrence			
IP:IV arm	0.75		
Patients alive (%)	45.4	53.6	
Overall survival			
Median (months)	52.2	63.2	0.05
Relative risk adjusted for survival			
IP:IV arm	0.78		

Table 4.3 Frequency of adverse events (grade ≥3) during any course of treatment on GOG 0114/SWOG 9227/ECOG-GO 114

Toxicity	IV cisplatin/IV paclitaxel ($n=227$)		Carboplatin/IP cisplatin/IV paclitaxel ($n=235$)	
	Grade 3 (%)	Grade 4 (%)	Grade 3 (%)	Grade 4 (%)
White blood cell count	49	13	49	28
Platelets	2	1	25	24
Gastrointestinal	9	8	17	20
Neurologic	8	<1	10	2

Adapted from Markman et al. [22]

Additionally, grade 3–4 gastrointestinal toxicity was also greater in patients receiving IP therapy; however, treatment-related death was equivalent between groups (two patients in each treatment arm).

Criticisms of GOG 0114/SWOG 9227/ECOG-GO 114 included the following: (1) the standard arm utilized IV cisplatin instead of IV carboplatin (i.e., results of GOG 0158 that were pivotal to the proof of IV carboplatin's superiority over IV cisplatin were not yet available); (2) the use in the experimental arm of two courses of moderately high-dose IV carboplatin before initiating the IP cisplatin/IV paclitaxel treatment gave platinum dose intensity and total dose advantages to the IP treatment regimen; and (3) since relatively severe myelosuppression was associated with the experimental regimen, it was concluded that it could not be considered standard-of-care, despite the more than 12-month survival advantage achieved in the patients randomized to the experimental IP/IV arm and the fact that the 5-year-median survival barrier finally had been overcome in patients with stage III, optimally resected ovarian cancer.

4.4
GOG 0172

Because of the controversy surrounding the design and toxicity associated with GOG-0114/SWOG 9227/ECOG-GO 114, GOG 0172 was developed as the penultimate phase III trial of IP vs. IV cisplatin, but in this case with the addition of IP paclitaxel in the experimental study arm. Because of the extremely advantageous pharmacokinetic profile of IP paclitaxel (i.e., IP/IV AUC concentration ratio of 800 to 1), the addition of IP paclitaxel on day 8 of a day 1 IV paclitaxel/day 2 IP cisplatin regimen was extremely attractive [7, 8]. In fact, a phase II trial of this regimen was piloted in the SWOG by Dr. Rothenberg and colleagues with good tolerance and a remarkably prolonged median progression-free survival of 33 months [14]. The schema for GOG 0172 is shown in Fig. 4.3. Again, patient eligibility was similar to that utilized in GOG 0104 and GOG 0114. The final results of this phase III trial of 415 randomized women with optimal, stage III disease were stunning; the IP to IV death hazard radio was 0.75 (95% CI, 0.58–0.97, $p=0.03$) [15]. The median survival was 49.7 and 65.6 months ($p=0.03$) and the median progression-free survival was 23.8 and 18.3 months for patients randomized to IV

Fig. 4.3 IV vs. IP/IV chemotherapy for stage III optimally, debulked ovarian cancer (GOG 0172) [15]

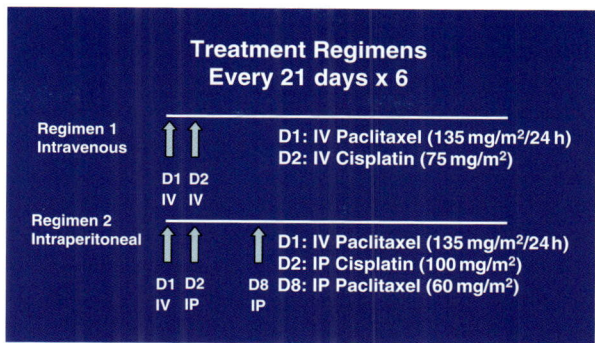

Table 4.4 Comparison of IP (GOG 0172) and IV (GOG 0158) therapy

Grade 3–4 toxicity	IP therapy (%)	IV therapy (%)
Leukopenia	76	59
Thrombocytopenia	12	39
Other hematologic	94[a]	90[b]
Gastrointestinal	46	10
Neurologic	19	7
Metabolic	27	2
Genitourinary	None reported	1
Pain	11	1
Catheter complications	19	N/A
Mean number of cycles completed	3.7	5.6

Adapted from Hess et al. [16]
[a]Primarily neutropenia and anemia
[b]Granulocytopenia only

or IP therapy, respectively. Since only 42% of the patients enrolled to the IP arm completed all six planned cycles of IP therapy, appropriate concern was raised regarding the tolerability of this regimen. Of interest, direct comparisons of the commonly used IV paclitaxel/IV carboplatin regimen from GOG 0158 to the IP regimen utilized in GOG 0172 suggests that the GOG 0172 IP/IV regimen may not be as difficult to tolerate as anticipated (Table 4.4) [16]. Of extreme relevance in this regard, Dr. Wenzel and colleagues performed a prospective quality-of-life analysis, using the functional assessment of cancer therapy (FACT) general and ovarian instruments. Twelve months postcycle 6, the patient-reported trial outcome index (TOI) scores obtained from the FACT were virtually identical for the IP and IV study groups [17].

The 16-month-median survival difference favoring the IP study arm of GOG 0172 (49.7 and 65.6 months for IV vs. IP therapy, respectively, $p=0.03$) was so compelling that the

NCI's division of cancer treatment and diagnosis (DCTD) issued a rare Clinical Announcement, along with a metaanalysis of IP vs. IV first-line phase III treatment studies in optimally debulked, stage III ovarian cancer [18]. The Clinical Announcement strongly stated that oncologists should discuss IP drug treatment options with all women who have stage III, minimal residual, optimally debulked epithelial ovarian cancer [18, 19]. The NCI-DCTD metaanalysis and our own more recent metaanalysis of the six IP cisplatin vs. IV studies, including 1,716 patients, showed an approximately 20% reduction in mortality associated with IP therapy (i.e., IP:IV death hazard ratio of 0.799, 95% CI, 0.702–0.910, $p=0.0007$) [18, 20, 21]. Furthermore, our pooled analyses of IP cisplatin-containing therapies suggest that other factors, such as IP catheter problems, cisplatin dose intensity, and the paclitaxel 24 h IV infusion, may have caused the drug intolerance observed in the GOG 0172 IP study group. Of importance, a pooled toxicity analysis of phase III trials of IP cisplatin vs. IV chemotherapy regimens documented that only gastrointestinal and febrile episodes were more common in the IP-treated patients. Conversely, ototoxicity was more common in IV treated patients (Table 4.5).

The Institute of Medicine, National Academy of Sciences, has defined the hierarchy of clinical trial evidence utilized to validate new, efficacious treatments in modern medicine. As shown in Fig. 4.4, the most convincing level of evidence is a metaanalysis of well-designed, well-powered, phase III clinical trials [21]. Thus far, there are at least three published metaanalyses concerning the efficacy of the IP route [18–21], all substantiating the clear survival benefit of cisplatin-based IP chemotherapy. The first of these metaanalyses appeared in the last week of December, 2005 as the primary component of a rare National Cancer Institute Clinical Announcement [18, 19]. The lead author, Edward Trimble, M.D., of NCI-DCTD-CTEP, and colleagues concluded that all women with stage III, optimally debulked ovarian cancer should be instructed about the potential benefits of IP-based regimen, based on the metaanalysis results that documented a pooled overall survival benefit to IP regimens (i.e., HR 0.79; 95% CI: 0.70–0.89), which almost exactly matched a pooled progression-free survival benefit (HR 0.79; 95% CI: 0.70–0.90) [18].

The two additional metaanalyses (i.e., unrelated to that published in 2006 online by Trimble et al, NCI-DCTD) have further documented the more than 20% risk reduction observed in both ovarian cancer recurrence and deaths associated with IP therapy, as

Table 4.5 Pooled ≥ grade 3 toxicity of IP cisplatin vs. IV regimens for advanced ovarian cancer

Toxicity	Odds ratio (95% CI)	p-Value
Leukopenia	1.07 (0.66–1.75)	NS
Hemoglobin	0.88 (0.58–1.35)	NS
Gastrointestinal	1.95 (1.17–3.240	0.01
Neurologic	1.22 (0.62–2.370	NS
Fever	1.7 (1.02–2.84)	0.04
Treatment-related death	1.4 (0.51–4.02)	NS
Ototoxicity	0.38 (0.19–0.73)	0.004

Adapted from Hess et al. [16]

Fig. 4.4 What is the level of clinical evidence?

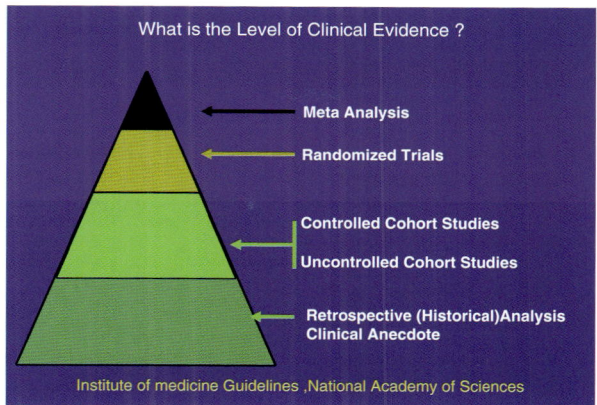

compared to intravenously administered drugs [20, 21]. In spite of the clarity of the National Institute of Medicine Grade A level of evidence for the substantial survival and progression-free survival benefits of IP chemotherapy, controversy continues about the phase III trials results. Listed in Table 4.6 are some of these arguments and counterpoints.

Clearly, IP cisplatin-containing therapy regimens offer significantly improved survival durations for women with stage III optimally debulked disease. The major toxicities associated with front-line cisplatin-based IP regimens remain grade 3–4 gastrointestinal (i.e., nausea, vomiting, abdominal pain) and grade 2–3 neurotoxicities (i.e., peripheral neuropathy); however, there is good reason to remain optimistic about our capability to both reduce their incidence and improve their treatment, as discussed later in this book. For example, the advent of longer acting 5HT3 inhibitors and central-acting antiemetics has greatly improved the control of these delayed onset cisplatin-associated toxicities. Furthermore, the reduction of the IP cisplatin dose to 75 mg/m^2 (i.e., 25% dose reduction) in most post-GOG 0172 regimens undoubtedly will reduce the incidence of peripheral neuropathy. It is essential to monitor the development of numbness and dysesthesia in fingers and toes and to discontinue or temporarily suspend IP cisplatin for grade 2 or greater neurotoxicity. It should be remembered that the prolonged survival on the IP arm of GOG 0172 (i.e., median of 65.9 months) was achieved, despite the fact that only 42% of the patients in the IP treatment group received six full cycles of IP therapy. This suggests that oncologists should feel justified in truncating the IP regimen at four or five cycles, in the setting of cumulative neurotoxicity of grade 2 or greater. There are putative agents for the prevention or amelioration of cisplatin- and/or paclitaxel-induced neurotoxicities, such as amifostine, gabapentin, glutamine, and l-carnitine, but none of these have been evaluated in the setting of well-powered, placebo-controlled randomized trials with patients undergoing IP/IV cisplatin-paclitaxel-based regimens. The GOG Cancer Prevention and Control Committee plans to initiate a phase III trial of l-carnitine vs. placebo within a fourth phase III IP therapy trial (i.e., GOG 0257). Additionally, there are plans for a pilot trial of orally-administered aprepitant for 6 days, rather than 3 days, combined in each case with long acting 5HT3 antiemetic regimens to prevent delayed nausea and vomiting, related to the GOG 0172 treatment regimen.

Table 4.6 Controversies concerning phase III IP/IV vs. IV chemotherapy GOG/SWOG/ECOG clinical trial results with corresponding counterpoints

Point	Counterpoint
Alberts et al. [10]	
IV cyclophosphamide no longer used in ovarian cancer treatment	This is not important since equal doses and identical schedules of IV and IP cisplatin were utilized
Patients with microscopic-only residual disease, at initial laparotomy, did not survive longer treated with IP, comparedto IV chemotherapy [10]	This was a secondary, add-on analysis of the trial. The validity of the surgical staging in this trial was upheld, in that patients with microscopic-only disease survived longest
IP/IV therapy too toxic [10]	In fact, IP/IV patients in this study experienced significantly less myelotoxicity, tinnitus, clinical hearing loss, and neurological complaints
Markman et al. [13]	
Patients in the IP/IV arm received two additional courses of upfront, IV medium high-dose carboplatin increasing platinum dose intensity)	In fact, the two upfront doses of carboplatin were likely detrimental in that 25% of the patients received either no IP cisplatin (i.e., 6.8%) or less than or equal to two cycles of IP cisplatin (i.e., 18.3%). Furthermore, several randomized trials have established that doubling the dose intensity of cisplatin or carboplatin results in increased toxicity, but no survival advantage in ovarian cancer [23, 24]
The IP/IV therapy was too myelotoxic and caused too much gastrointestinal toxicity [12]	In fact, the myelotoxicity associated with the IP/IV regimen was more related to the IV carboplatin therapy component, and the gastrointestinal toxicity was relatively short-lived. Furthermore, toxicity-related deaths were equivalent in the two study arms
Armstrong [15]	
Because the GOG 0172 experimental regimen was so intolerable, it cannot be used as a standard therapy for stage III minimal residual disease [15]	In fact, a careful quality-of-life evaluation using the FACT-0 tool showed 12 months postcompletion of all chemotherapy in GOG-0172, equivalent quality-of-life indices data for both the control and experimental treatment patient groups [17]
Metaanalyses, Trimble et al. [19], Jaaback [21], Hess et al. [20]	
These metaanalyses were weighted mainly by the three U.S. GOG Intergroup studies [20, 21]	The results of the three different metaanalyses performed by biostatisticians and healthcare outcomes experts document the increased efficacy for IP therapy. None of the metaanalyses excluded the trials of international groups and weighting techniques account for sample size differences. The largest trials of IP therapy were conducted in the U.S.

Table 4.6 (continued)

Point	Counterpoint
Armstrong et al. [15]	
IV cisplatin/IV paclitaxel was the wrong control arm [15]	In fact, NCI mandated this as the control arm because the results of GOG 0158 (i.e., IV cisplatin/IV paclitaxel vs. IV carboplatin/IV paclitaxel) were not available; however, GOG 0158 did not document a survival advantage for the carboplatin arm [12]
The extra dose of day 8 IP paclitaxel gave unfair advantage to the IP arm	Granted that weekly IV paclitaxel appears more active than every 3 week paclitaxel; the day 8 dosing design was the design that was piloted in phase I and II IP/IV studies in the SWOG [14]
Only 42% of patients on the IP study arm completed the planned six cycles of IP/IV therapy, because of drug toxicity, IP catheter dysfunction, etc., additional insight concerning the impact of IP chemotherapy [15]	In spite of the fact that less than 50% of patients on the IP arm received less than six cycles of IP/IV GOG 0172 experimental arm therapy, there still was a 16-month survival advantage for the IP/IV study arm. Perhaps no more than four cycles are necessary to convey the survival advantage

4.5
Future Phase III IP Trials

The GOG is conducting a phase III follow-up study to GOG 0172, which is being designed to answer multiple questions, including:

- The efficacy of a revised GOG 0172 regimen, to reduce both myelotoxicity (i.e., switch from the day 1, 24 h paclitaxel IV infusion to the 3 h infusion) and neurotoxicity (i.e., decrease IP cisplatin dose to 75 mg/m^2 on day 2).
- The comparative activity of IP and IV carboplatin, as well as IP carboplatin compared to IP cisplatin when combined with weekly paclitaxel.
- The efficacy of an IV carboplatin, weekly IV paclitaxel plus IV bevacizumab regimen compared to the IP carboplatin and IP cisplatin regimens, also combined with IV bevacizumab every 3 weeks for six courses.

The schema for GOG 0252 is shown in Fig. 4.5. As shown, eligibility is similar to the prior three phase III IP trials, involving previously untreated patients with stage III, minimal residual disease, epithelial-type ovarian cancer (excluding clear cell carcinomas). It is an important interesting trial that will enroll women to one of three treatment arms. Participants enrolled to arm number one will receive IV carboplatin (AUC=6 mg min/mL) on day 1 plus IV paclitaxel 75/m^2 on days 1 and 8 plus IV bevacizumab, 15 mg/kg IV day 1 with cycles repeated every 21 days. Arm two of this trial will evaluate the comparative

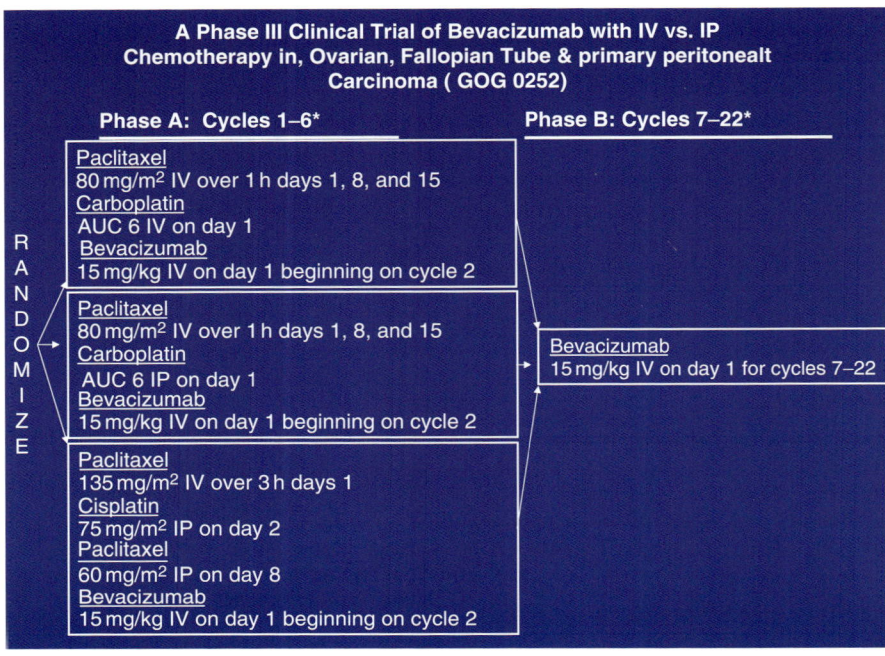

Fig. 4.5 A phase III clinical trial of bevacizumab with IV vs. IP chemotherapy in, ovarian, fallopian tube and primary peritoneal carcinoma (GOG-0252)

activity of IP carboplatin (AUC=6 mg min/mL) on day 1 plus IV paclitaxel 75 mg/m² on days 1 and 8 plus IV bevacizumab 15 mg/kg on day 1 of each 21 day cycle. Finally, arm three will test the revised GOG 0172 IP/IV regimen, including IP cisplatin 75 mg/m² on day 1 plus IV paclitaxel 135 mg/m² on day 2 over 3 h and IP paclitaxel 60 mg/m² on day 8 plus IV bevacizumab 15 mg/kg on day 1 of every 21 day cycle.

4.6
Conclusion

There are very few clinical research experiences in oncology, which have yielded such consistent findings as have the phase III trials of IP vs. IV chemotherapy for stage III, minimal residual disease ovarian cancer. The data document a one-to-one and a half-year survival advantage for simply administering active drugs, such as cisplatin and paclitaxel, into the IP space as compared to exclusively IV delivery. The evidence from at least three well-performed and published metaanalyses provide Grade A evidence (Institute of Medicine Guidelines) of the efficacy of IP therapy for stage III minimal residual disease [18–21]. Clearly, as stated in a 2006 NCI-DCDT-CTEP clinical announcement, women with optimally debulked, stage III ovarian cancer must be informed about the benefits of

IP therapy. Nevertheless, there are many unanswered questions concerning the future development of regional therapy for these women, which should be answered if we are to see further survival and quality-of-life improvements. These include the following:

- Can the efficacy of the GOG 0172 regimen be preserved as its myelotoxicity and neurotoxicity potentials are reduced through reductions of IP cisplatin dosing to 75 mg/m^2 and IV paclitaxel infusion to 3 h [15]?
- Can IP carboplatin replace IP cisplatin while preserving the survival advantage of the latter and the reduced neurotoxicity and gastrointestinal side effects of the former?
- Can bevacizumab be safely and effectively added to the IP platinum/IP-IV paclitaxel regimens?
- Will the addition of bevacizumab result in prolonged progression-free and overall survivals (as compared to historical data generated by Dr. Armstrong and colleagues) [15]?
- Are there other cytotoxic and/or biological agents that could be added to present IP/IV drug regimens to improve efficacy (e.g., IP pemetrexed or IV pertuzimab)?
- Can supportive care therapy be improved to reduce the neurotoxicity (e.g., l-carnitine, glutamine) and gastrointestinal toxicity (e.g., 6-day aprepitant vs. 3-day aprepitant schedules) associated with the GOG 0172 regimen [15]?
- Can we determine the best IP catheters to reduce fibroblast sheath formation, catheter dysfunction, and small bowel obstruction or perforation?

It is time to understand that the IP route of therapy for stage III, minimal residual ovarian cancer is now established as a standard therapeutic approach for the care of women diagnosed with this disease. We should resolve the controversies through the use of well-designed phase III clinical trials, extending patient accrual to all cooperative groups, both in the U.S. and internationally.

References

1. Dedrick RL et al (1978) Pharmacokinetic rationale for peritoneal drug administration in the treatment of ovarian cancer. Cancer Treat Rep 62(1):1–11
2. Speyer JL, Myers CE (1980) The use of peritoneal dialysis for delivery of chemotherapy to intraperitoneal malignancies. Recent Results Cancer Res 74:264–269
3. Speyer JL et al (1980) Phase I and pharmacological studies of 5-fluorouracil administered intraperitoneally. Cancer Res 40(3):567–572
4. Casper ES et al (1983) Ip cisplatin in patients with malignant ascites: pharmacokinetic evaluation and comparison with the iv route. Cancer Treat Rep 67(3):235–238
5. Howell SB et al (1982) Intraperitoneal cisplatin with systemic thiosulfate protection. Ann Intern Med 97(6):845–851
6. Howell SB et al (1987) Long-term survival of advanced refractory ovarian carcinoma patients with small-volume disease treated with intraperitoneal chemotherapy. J Clin Oncol 5(10): 1607–1612

7. Francis P et al (1995) Phase I feasibility and pharmacologic study of weekly intraperitoneal paclitaxel: a Gynecologic Oncology Group pilot study. J Clin Oncol 13(12):2961–2967
8. Markman M et al (1992) Phase I trial of intraperitoneal taxol: a Gynecologic Oncology Group study. J Clin Oncol 10(9):1485–1491
9. Muggia FM et al (1996) Intraperitoneal mitoxantrone or floxuridine: effects on time-to-failure and survival in patients with minimal residual ovarian cancer after second-look laparotomy – a randomized phase II study by the Southwest Oncology Group. Gynecol Oncol 61(3): 395–402
10. Alberts DS et al (1996) Intraperitoneal cisplatin plus intravenous cyclophosphamide versus intravenous cisplatin plus intravenous cyclophosphamide for stage III ovarian cancer. N Engl J Med 335(26):1950–1955
11. Alberts DS et al (1992) Improved therapeutic index of carboplatin plus cyclophosphamide versus cisplatin plus cyclophosphamide: final report by the Southwest Oncology Group of a phase III randomized trial in stages III and IV ovarian cancer. J Clin Oncol 10(5):706–717
12. Ozols RF et al (2003) Phase III trial of carboplatin and paclitaxel compared with cisplatin and paclitaxel in patients with optimally resected stage III ovarian cancer: a Gynecologic Oncology Group study. J Clin Oncol 21(17):3194–3200
13. Markman M et al (2001) Phase III trial of standard-dose intravenous cisplatin plus paclitaxel versus moderately high-dose carboplatin followed by intravenous paclitaxel and intraperitoneal cisplatin in small-volume stage III ovarian carcinoma: an intergroup study of the Gynecologic Oncology Group, Southwestern Oncology Group, and Eastern Cooperative Oncology Group. J Clin Oncol 19(4):1001–1007
14. Rothenberg ML et al (2003) Combined intraperitoneal and intravenous chemotherapy for women with optimally debulked ovarian cancer: results from an intergroup phase II trial. J Clin Oncol 21(7):1313–1319
15. Armstrong DK et al (2006) Intraperitoneal cisplatin and paclitaxel in ovarian cancer. N Engl J Med 354(1):34–43
16. Hess LH, Chambers SK, Alberts DS (2008) Role of intraperitoneal chemotherapy for ovarian cancer. In: DeVita VT Jr, Lawrence TS, Rosenberg SA (eds) Cancer principles and practice of oncology. Wolters Kluwer Health, Inc, New York
17. Wenzel LB et al (2007) Health-related quality of life during and after intraperitoneal versus intravenous chemotherapy for optimally debulked ovarian cancer: a Gynecologic Oncology Group study. J Clin Oncol 25(4):437–443
18. Trimble EL, Christian MC (2006) Intraperitoneal chemotherapy for women with advanced epithelial ovarian carcinoma. Gynecol Oncol 100(1):3–4
19. Trimble EL, Alvarez RD (2006) Intraperitoneal chemotherapy and the NCI clinical announcement. Gynecol Oncol 103(2 suppl 1):S18–S19
20. Hess LM et al (2007) A meta-analysis of the efficacy of intraperitoneal cisplatin for the frontline treatment of ovarian cancer. Int J Gynecol Cancer 17(3):561–570
21. Jaaback K, Johnson N (2006) Intraperitoneal chemotherapy for the initial management of primary epithelial ovarian cancer (review). Cochrane Database Syst Rev 25; (1): CD 005340
22. Markman M et al (1992) Impact on survival of surgically defined favorable responses to salvage intraperitoneal chemotherapy in small-volume residual ovarian cancer. J Clin Oncol 10(9):1479–1484
23. Gore M et al (1998) Randomized trial of dose-intensity with single-agent carboplatin in patients with epithelial ovarian cancer. London Gynaecological Oncology Group. J Clin Oncol 16(7):2426–2434
24. McGuire WP et al (1995) Assessment of dose-intensive therapy in suboptimally debulked ovarian cancer: a Gynecologic Oncology Group study. J Clin Oncol 13(7):1589–1599

Criteria for Using Intraperitoneal (IP) Chemotherapy for Advanced Ovarian Cancer

5

Richard R. Barakat

5.1
Frontline Therapy

5.1.1
Impact of the Size of Residual Disease

Ovarian cancer is a disease that remains confined to the abdominal cavity in the majority of cases. IP therapy, therefore, offers an attractive treatment strategy for providing high concentrations of drugs directly to tumor sites. The size of any remaining tumor nodules at the initiation of chemotherapy is the most critical factor in selecting patients who may benefit from IP therapy. It has been demonstrated that chemotherapeutic agents can penetrate into tumor nodules approximately 1–2 mm from the surface. Then, theoretically, IP therapy should only benefit patients with very small residual disease at the initiation of therapy or it must be combined with intravenous therapy that can reach the center of tumor nodules. Los et al. [1] used an IP rat model to demonstrate that the concentration of cisplatin was higher in the periphery of tumor nodules following IP administration, while the concentration in the center was equivalent to that of intravenously (IV) administered cisplatin. By convention, optimal residual disease is defined as no individual tumor mass greater than 1 cm in diameter. Most recent trials of IP therapy include this definition as part of their eligibility criteria. Whether or not patients with larger disease at the initiation of IP therapy may also benefit from IP therapy is controversial. GOG 0104, a randomized trial of IV cyclophosphamide plus IP cipslatin vs. IV cylophosphamide plus IV cisplatin [2], permitted accrual of women with residual disease up to 2 cm in diameter. The effect of the treatment route (IV vs. IP) was not influenced by the size of the residual disease (microscopic vs. ≤0.5 cm vs. >0.5–2 cm). Although it is possible that women with suboptimal disease may benefit from IP therapy, the majority of randomized trials that have demonstrated a benefit to IP therapy have included patients with optimal residual disease [3, 4].

R.R. Barakat
Department of Surgery, Memorial Sloan-Kettering Cancer Center,
1274 York Avenue, New York, NY 10065, USA
e-mail: gynbreast@mskcc.org

D.S. Alberts et al. (eds.), *Intraperitoneal Therapy for Ovarian Cancer*,
DOI: 10.1007/978-3-642-12130-2_5, © Springer-Verlag Berlin Heidelberg 2010

5.1.2
Impact of Chemical Debulking Prior to IP Therapy

It has been hypothesized that employing systemically administered cytotoxic agents to chemically debulk residual cancer before regional drug delivery will optimize the benefits of IP therapy by reducing the size of any residual tumor nodules to less than that which can be accomplished surgically [5]. A trial was conducted at Memorial Sloan-Kettering to study the effect of intensified intravenous cyclophosphamide/cisplatin and interim surgical debulking followed by IP cisplatin on surgically defined complete remission rate and survival in advanced ovarian cancer. Following an initial laparotomy for diagnosis and debulking, 36 patients with stage IIB - IV ovarian cancer received two cycles, spaced 28 days apart, of intravenous cisplatin 30–40 $mg/m^2/day$ with hypertonic saline for 4–5 days and cyclophosphamide 200 $mg/m^2/day$ for 5 days. A second laparotomy was done to further debulk the remaining cancer and to place an IP catheter. Four cycles of IP cisplatin at 50 or 100 mg/m^2 were administered 21 days apart followed by a third laparotomy to define response and plan any further therapy. The surgically confirmed complete response rate was 47% and median survival was 68.3 months. Ten of the 17 patients (58.8%) relapsed following complete response at a median of 19.5 months (range, 5–98). Both aggressive chemotherapy and surgery seemed to play a role in inducing this high complete response rate. Traditional prognostic factors, including the stage and the diameter of the largest residual disease, had little apparent effect on the likelihood of complete response or survival, whereas tumor grade had a more significant effect on survival. Neurotoxicity was dose limiting. The high complete response rate achieved in this trial suggests that the multimodality approach of up-front debulking with intravenous chemotherapy followed by interval surgical debulking and IP cisplatin is worthy of further study. The high relapse rate among complete responders and the unacceptable neurotoxicity also suggest that modifications could improve the results.

To test the potential clinical advantage of combining systemic chemical debulking with IP cisplatin in patients also receiving IV-administered paclitaxel, the Gynecologic Oncology Group (GOG), Southwest Oncology Group (SWOG), and the Eastern Cooperative Oncology Group (ECOG) initiated a randomized controlled phase III trial of standard-dose IV cisplatin/paclitaxel for six courses, compared with an experimental regimen of two cycles of moderately high-dose single-agent carboplatin, area under curve (AUC) 9, followed by six courses of IP cisplatin and IV paclitaxel [4]. Patients with optimally debulked (≤ 1 cm residual) cancer were randomized to receive either IV paclitaxel 135 mg/m^2 over 24 h followed by IV cisplatin 75 mg/m^2 every 3 weeks for six courses or IV carboplatin (AUC 9) every 28 days for two courses, then IV paclitaxel 135 mg/m^2 over 24 h followed by IP cisplatin 100 mg/m^2 every 3 weeks for six courses. Of the 523 patients who entered this trial, 462 were determined to be assessable, with prognostic factors well balanced between the treatments. Neutropenia, thrombocytopenia, and gastrointestinal and metabolic toxicities were greater in the experimental arm. As a result, 18% of the patients received less than two courses of IP therapy. Progression-free survival was superior for patients randomized to the experimental treatment arm (median, 28 vs. 22 months; relative risk, 0.78; log-rank $p=0.01$). There was a borderline improvement in overall survival associated with this regimen (median, 63 vs. 52 months; relative risk, 0.81; $p=0.05$). The authors concluded that "chemical debulking" with an experimental regimen including moderately high-dose IV carboplatin followed by IP paclitaxel and IV cisplatin yielded a significant improvement in progression-free survival when compared with a standard regimen of IV cisplatin and paclitaxel. Because the improvement in overall survival was of borderline statistical significance and the toxicity was greater, the experimental arm is not recommended for routine use. However, the results provided direction for further clinical investigation of IP therapy in small-volume ovarian cancer whether achieved by surgical or chemical debulking.

5.1.3
Impact of Disease Stage

Little is known about IP therapy for patients with stage IV disease, and no data comparing the different subsets of stage IV diseases with regard to the site of extraperitoneal disease and IP therapy are available. Up-front IP therapy in optimally debulked patients with stage IV epithelial ovarian cancer (EOC) is controversial since the anticipated added benefit derived from enhanced drug exposure is not thought to be applicable to extraperitoneal sites. Many practitioners will not offer up-front IP therapy to patients with optimally debulked stage IV disease since there has been no demonstrated proven benefit in randomized phase III trials for this group of patients.

5.2
Consolidation Therapy

5.2.1
Consolidation Therapy for Patients with no Residual Disease

In addition to the frontline therapy for optimally debulked ovarian cancer, IP chemotherapy has been investigated as a consolidation therapy after a negative second-look reassessment, and as second-line treatment for persistent disease. Barakat et al. evaluated the efficacy of three courses of IP cisplatin (CDDP) and etoposide (VP-16) as a consolidation therapy following pathologically negative second-look surgical reassessment for Stage IIC-IV EOC [6]. Between September 1988 and April 1996, 40 patients were treated with three cycles of IP CDDP (100 mg/m^2)/VP-16 (200 mg/m^2) as a consolidation therapy. Survival was compared to that of a group of 46 contemporaneous patients matched for stage, grade, age, and size of the residual disease who were undergoing observation only upon completion of initial surgery. With a median follow-up of 36 months in both groups, 14/36 (39%) of the protocol group recurred, compared with 25/46 (54%) of those undergoing observation alone. Median disease-free survival (DFS) for the observed patients was 28.5 months, a DFS which had not been reached in the consolidation group. DFS distribution between the two groups was compared using the log-rank test and was found to be significant ($p = 0.03$). Multivariate analysis revealed that the only significant predictor of improved DFS was protocol treatment ($p < 0.01$). The authors concluded that the use of IP consolidation with CDDP/VP-16 following negative second-look reassessment in patients with advanced EOC resulted in a significant increase in DFS compared to nonprotocol patients treated concurrently who underwent observation alone. However, in one of the few published randomized trials of IP consolidation therapy following a negative second-look procedure, the European Organization for Research and Treatment of Cancer (EORTC) enrolled 153 pathologically complete responders following platinum-based systemic chemotherapy. The 8-year progression-free survival and 8-year overall survival were similar in patients who received IP CDDP 90 mg/m^2 every 3 weeks for four cycles and in those who had no further treatment after second-look surgery (38 vs. 37 and 53 vs. 48%, respectively; p=NS) [7].

5.2.2
Consolidation Therapy for Patients with Minimal Residual Disease

Randomized trials evaluating IP therapy as an initial treatment for advanced EOC have been conducted, but no randomized data evaluating IP therapy as a consolidation or second-line therapy for the treatment of persistent disease are available. Previously reported data from multiple phase II trials in patients with small-volume (<1 cm residual) disease treated with various platinum-containing regimens have indicated surgical response rates of 40–50% and surgical complete response rates of 25–35% [8]. Barakat et al. [8] reviewed the MSKCC experience with 433 patients who received IP therapy between 1984 and 1998 following debulking surgery and IV chemotherapy either as a consolidation or as a treatment for persistent disease. The median survival from the initiation of IP therapy by the size of the residual disease was none, 8.7 years; microscopic, 4.8 years; less than 1 cm, 3.3 years; more than 1 cm, 1.2 years. In a multivariate analysis, the only significant predictors of long-term survival were tumor grade and the size of the residual disease at the initiation of IP therapy. The authors concluded that prolonged survival was observed in selected patients receiving IP platinum-based therapy. Although it was impossible to determine the exact contribution of IP therapy to survival in this study, a clear relationship between the size of the disease at the initiation of IP therapy and the long-term survival was demonstrated.

5.2.3
Impact of Retroperitoneal Disease

The retroperitoneal nodes are involved in up to 80% of patients with advanced EOC. It is unclear as to whether or not these nodes represent a sanctuary for cancer cells that were not removed at initial surgery. Barakat et al. [9] evaluated the impact of retroperitoneal lymph node disease on the efficacy of salvage IP therapy. They retrospectively reviewed 41 patients with advanced EOC treated between 9/83 and 7/95 who had undergone retroperitoneal nodal sampling prior to salvage IP therapy. Of the 41 patients, 19 (46%) were noted to have disease involving retroperitoneal nodes at initial surgery or at reassessment laparotomy, while 22 (54%) had biopsy-proven negative nodes. All the patients were treated with salvage IP therapy. With a median follow-up of 26 months since surgical reassessment, the median survival in the node-positive group was 31 months, which was not significantly different from the node negative group. This led the authors to conclude that the presence of disease in the retroperitoneal nodes was not a contraindication for the use of salvage IP chemotherapy for patients with advanced EOC.

5.2.4
Impact of Stage IV Disease

Studies investigating the use of IP chemotherapy in patients with stage III and IV EOC after second-look assessment have noted prolonged survival in select patients with minimal residual disease at the time of second-look assessment [8, 10, 11]. Zivanovic et al. evaluated overall survival in patients with stage IV EOC treated with IP chemotherapy after second-look assessment following frontline IV therapy between 1984 and 1998 [12]. Within the group of patients with stage IV disease, they also sought to determine how the outcome was affected by the site of metastasis and considered this in relation to Stage III disease. Second-look assessments were performed both via laparotomy and laparoscopy. Overall survival was defined as the interval between second-look surgery and death or last follow-up. The median survival of patients with stage IIIC disease was significantly better (42 vs. 34 months) than that of patients with stage IV disease. The only significant predictor of survival in patients with stage IV disease treated with IP therapy was the presence of gross residual disease at the initiation of IP therapy. Median survival for those with stage IV and no gross residual disease prior to the initiation of IP therapy was 38 months, compared to 18 months for those with gross residual disease. The site of stage IV disease was also an important predictor of survival. The median survival for stage IV patients with malignant pleural effusions only was better (38 months) than that of patients with other stage IV disease (25 months), but this did not reach statistical significance. Ten stage IV patients (20%) survived more than 5 years. In this series, patients with stage IV disease who were treated with primary cytoreduction and intravenous chemotherapy and were subsequently treated with IP therapy had a better median overall survival if no gross residual disease was found at second-look reassessment. Drugs delivered by the IP route penetrate only a depth of a few millimeters beneath the tumor surface [1, 13, 14]. Thus, patients with small-volume residual disease benefit the most from this approach. Although randomized trials evaluating the role of consolidation strategies have not demonstrated a statistically significant improvement of overall survival, they have suggested that these strategies are most effective for patients who have responded to primary therapy [15–19]. Undoubtedly, there are methodological issues that may not permit the generalization of these findings to contemporary patients. The heterogeneity of treatment strategies throughout the study period makes it difficult to account for the differences in treatment regimens used during and after IP consolidation therapy. These findings are also limited by a long study period. During this time period, both the standard chemotherapy agents and surgical techniques have improved. Cyclophosphamide and cisplatin are no longer the standard agents used for treating primary EOC. Surgical technique, instrumentation, and approach have all improved as evidenced by the current optimal cytoreduction rate at this institution, which is nearly 80%, compared to only 37% in the reported series [20].

In conclusion, the survival of patients diagnosed with stage IV EOC continues to be short, and even in this "favorable" group selected for IP therapy after achieving a clinical remission, only two patients survived. While new approaches are undoubtedly needed, identification of a group of patients with stage IV disease who may benefit from IP consolidation is warranted. Optimal cytoreduction rates may prove helpful in enhancing the survival rates even for stage IV patients, and certain subsets may benefit from the implementation of strategies heretofore thought to be applicable only to stage III patients. Since all stage IV patients receive intravenous therapy, consolidation IP therapy may offer an opportunity to extend the benefits of the IP route to a population with a historically poor outcome.

5.2.5
Presence of Adhesions

One possible explanation for the failure of the high concentrations of cytotoxic agents achieved following IP drug delivery to produce a favorable response in patients with ovarian cancer is the inability of the drug-containing fluid to be adequately distributed throughout the peritoneal cavity. This is usually due to intraabdominal adhesion formation. To evaluate the influence of the severity of adhesions on the ability to achieve a surgically defined complete response (S-CR), Markman et al. [21] retrospectively reviewed the operative reports of 70 patients with small-volume residual ovarian cancer treated on one of the three Phase II salvage IP trials at the Memorial Sloan-Kettering Cancer Center. Adhesions were observed at the time of laparotomy performed immediately preceding the initiation of IP therapy, The S-CR rate in the 36 patients with limited adhesion formation observed upon entering the peritoneal cavity was 28%, compared to 35% in the 34 patients with extensive adhesions ($p \geq 0.05$). In 33 patients treated with a phase-2 cisplatin-based IP program, who had previously responded to systemic platinum, 47% (8/17) and 44% (7/16) of those with limited and extensive adhesions, respectively, achieved a S-CR ($p > 0.05$). Markman et al. concluded that the presence of extensive adhesions observed within the peritoneal cavity at the time of a laparotomy performed immediately prior to the initiation of IP therapy does not have a negative impact on the potential to achieve an S-CR, assuming that it is technically feasible to lyse all significant adhesions prior to the completion of the operative procedure.

5.3
Conclusions

The unique pattern of IP spread for EOC makes this disease ideally suited for IP chemotherapy, a mode of delivery in which high concentrations of drugs can be introduced directly to tumor sites. The size of any remaining tumor nodules at the initiation of chemotherapy is the critical factor in selecting patients who may benefit from IP therapy. Although it has been demonstrated that chemotherapeutic agents can penetrate into tumor nodules approximately 1–2 mm from the surface, phase III clinical trials have demonstrated a benefit to IP therapy in patients with residual disease up to 2 cm. The preponderance of evidence from phase III clinical trials, however, would indicate that in the up-front setting, IP therapy should be reserved for those with optimal residual disease (defined as no tumor that is greater than 1 cm in diameter remaining after surgery). The same holds true for patients receiving IP therapy in the consolidation or second-line setting, where the greatest benefit is for patients with microscopic residual disease following IP therapy, followed by those with residual disease ≤1 cm in diameter. The retroperitoneal nodes have been considered a sanctuary for tumor cells, and the presence of metastatic disease in these nodes may represent a contraindication to IP therapy. The data available on this topic are limited, but one small retrospective study reported that the presence of metastatic disease in retroperitoneal nodes did not appear to be a contraindication to IP therapy. Finally, patients with persistent stage IV disease may benefit from IP therapy, especially if they have no gross residual disease following initial therapy and were considered stage IV based on pleural effusion alone. There is no data on the role of up-front IP therapy in those patients with stage IV disease at initial presentation.

References

1. Los G, Mutsaers PH, van der Vijgh WJ et al (1989) Direct diffusion of cisdiamminedichloroplatinum (II) in intraperitoneal rat tumors after intraperitoneal chemotherapy: a comparison with systemic chemotherapy. Cancer Res 49:3380–3384
2. Alberts DS, Liu PY, Hannigan EV et al (1996) Intraperitoneal cisplatin plus intravenous cyclophosphamide versus intravenous cisplatin plus intravenous cyclophosphamide for stage III ovarian cancer. N Engl J Med 335:1950–1955
3. Armstrong DK, Bundy B, Wenzel L et al (2006) Intraperitoneal cisplatin and paclitaxel in ovarian cancer. N Engl J Med 354:34–43
4. Markman M, Bundy BN, Alberts DS et al (2001) Phase III trial of standard-dose intravenous cisplatin plus paclitaxel and intraperitoneal cisplatin in small-volume stage III ovarian carcinoma: an intergroup study of the Gynecologic Oncology Group, Southwestern Oncology Group, and Eastern Cooperative Oncology Group. J Clin Oncol 19:1001–1007
5. Shapiro F, Schneider J, Markman MM et al (1997) High-intensity intravenous cyclophosphamide and cisplatin, interim surgical debulking, and intraperitoneal cisplatin in advanced ovarian carcinoma: a pilot trial with ten-year follow-up. Gynecol Oncol 67:39–45
6. Barakat RR, Almadrones L, Venkatraman ES et al (1998) A phase II trial of intraperitoneal cisplatin and etoposide as consolidation therapy in patients with Stage II-IV epithelial ovarian cancer following negative surgical assessment. Gynecol Oncol 69:17–22
7. Piccart MJ, Floquet A, Scarfone G et al (2003) Intraperitoneal cisplatin versus no further treatment: 8-year results of EORTC 55875, a randomized phase III study in ovarian cancer patients with a pathologically complete remission after platinum-based intravenous chemotherapy. Int J Gynecol Cancer 13:196–203
8. Barakat RR, Sabbatini P, Bhaskaran D et al (2002) Intraperitoneal chemotherapy for ovarian carcinoma: results of long-term follow-up. J Clin Oncol 20:694–698
9. Barakat RR, Fennelly D, Pizzuto F, Venkatraman ES, Brown C, Curtin JP (1997) Salvage intraperitoneal therapy of advanced epithelial ovarian cancer: impact of retroperitoneal nodal disease. Eur J Gynaecol Oncol 18:161–163
10. Sabbatini P, Spriggs DR (2006) Consolidation for ovarian cancer in remission. J Clin Oncol 24:537–539
11. Tournigarnd C, Louvet C, Molitor JL et al (2003) Long-term survival with consolidation intraperitoneal chemotherapy for patients with advanced ovarian cancer with pathological complete remission. Gynecol Oncol 91:341–345

12. Zivanovic O, Barakat RR, Sabbatini PJ et al (2008) Prognostic factors for patients with stage IV epithelial ovarian cancer receiving intraperitoneal chemotherapy after second-look assessment: results of long-term follow-up. Cancer 112:2690–2697

13. Los G, Mutsaers PH, Lenglet WJ, Baldew GS, McVie JG (1990) Platinum distribution in intraperitoneal tumors after intraperitoneal cisplatin treatment. Cancer Chemother Pharmacol 25:389–394

14. Los G, Verdegaal EM, Mutsaers PH, McVie JG (1991) Penetration of carboplatin and cisplatin into rat peritoneal tumor nodules after intraperitoneal chemotherapy. Cancer Chemother Pharmacol 28:159–165

15. Berek JS, Taylor PT, Gordon A et al (2004) Randomized, placebo controlled study of oregovomab for consolidation of clinical remission in patients with advanced ovarian cancer. J Clin Oncol 22:3507–3516

16. Markman M (2003) Rationale for maintenance or consolidation therapy in ovarian cancer. Clin Adv Hematol Oncol 1:176–178

17. Markman M (2003) Consolidation/maintenance chemotherapy for ovarian cancer. Curr Oncol Rep 5:454–458

18. Markman M, Liu PY, Wilczynski S et al (2003) Southwest Oncology Group; Gynecologic Oncology Group. Phase III randomized trial of 12 versus 3 months of maintenance paclitaxel in patients with advanced ovarian cancer after complete response to platinum and paclitaxel-based chemotherapy: a Southwest Oncology Group and Gynecologic Oncology Group trial. J Clin Oncol 21:2460–2465

19. Nicholson S, Gooden CS, Hird V et al (1998) Radioimmunotherapy after chemotherapy compared to chemotherapy alone in the treatment of advanced ovarian cancer: a matched analysis. Oncol Rep 5:223–226

20. Chi DS, Franklin CC, Levine DA et al (2004) Improved optimal cytoreduction rates for stages IIIC and IV epithelial ovarian, fallopian tube, and primary peritoneal cancer: a change in surgical approach. Gynecol Oncol 94:650–654

21. Markman M, Jones W, Lewis JL Jr et al (1992) Impact of laparotomy finding of significant intrabdominal adhesions on the surgically defined complete response rate to subsequent salvage intraperitoneal chemotherapy. J Cancer Res Clin Oncol 118:163–165

Selection and Placement of Intraperitoneal Catheters for IP Chemotherapy for Ovarian Cancer

6

Joan Walker

6.1
Introduction

Despite the publication of the landmark randomized clinical trial by the Gynecologic Oncology Group (GOG) in January 2006 [1], GOG 0172, with paclitaxel 135 mg/m^2 intravenous (IV) over 24 h, followed on day 2 with cisplatin 100 mg/m^2 IP, and day 8 paclitaxel 60 mg/m^2 IP, showing a significant improvement in survival over a cisplatin/paclitaxel intravenous approach, IP therapy has not gained widespread acceptance by the oncology community. The remarkable overall median survival of 65.6 months was 16 months longer among women randomized to IP treatment as compared to the IV control. It appears that the toxicity, and difficulty in administering the IP regimen, outweighs any survival benefit in the minds of treating oncologists. The appropriate drugs, doses, schedule, and indications for intraperitoneal chemotherapy, remain areas of controversy since the publication. In order for IP therapy to become implemented nationwide, there is a need to establish a regimen with acceptable toxicity and ease of administration, which preserves the survival advantage. It is important to remember that GOG 0172 administered 100 mg/m^2 of cisplatin IP from March 1998 through January of 2001, when odansetron was very expensive and therefore not available to many patients, and aprepitant was not approved by the United States Food and Drug Administration (FDA). Generic odansetron was available in 2006, oral aprepitant was approved in 2003, and the IV formulation became available in 2008. The availability of these new antiemetics, aggressive intravenous saline hydration, and supportive care strategies allow for the safe administration of a high dose of IP cisplatin in an outpatient setting in the majority of patients [2–4]. Peripheral neuropathy, however, remains an unresolved issue at these doses [5].

Looking into the future of IP chemotherapy, we must understand what has transpired since the publication of the GOG 0172 IP regimen in 2006. In an attempt to optimize the IP regimen and make it acceptable to patients and oncologists by improving the ease of administration, decreasing toxicity, and preserving survival, the following issues were

J. Walker
Department of Obstetrics and Gynecology, University of Oklahoma Health Science Center,
P.O. Box 26001, Oklahoma, OK 73104, USA
e-mail: Joan-walker@ouhsc.edu

D.S. Alberts et al. (eds.), *Intraperitoneal Therapy for Ovarian Cancer*,
DOI: 10.1007/978-3-642-12130-2_6, © Springer-Verlag Berlin Heidelberg 2010

considered by the GOG: (1) the benefit vs. toxicity of day 8 IP paclitaxel; (2) the toxicity differences of IP delivery of cisplatin on the day following the paclitaxel compared to the convenience of same day administration; (3) the toxicity and efficacy of reducing the cisplatin dose; (4) the toxicity benefit vs. the potential reduced disease free interval with IP carboplatin [2] compared to IP cisplatin; and (5) outpatient administration benefits of a 3-h infusion of paclitaxel.

Valid concerns about neurotoxicity are raised by reducing the paclitaxel infusion to 3 h and giving the IP cisplatin on the same day in an outpatient setting [6, 7]. A paclitaxel infusion of 175 mg/m^2 over 3 h has been shown to be equivalent to a 24-h paclitaxel infusion of 135 mg/m^2 in platinum regimens [7], although there is increased neurotoxicity with the addition of cisplatin, especially when given on the same day. However, giving cisplatin via the IP route on the same day may prove acceptable and tolerable since systemic absorption of cisplatin is delayed due to the pharmacokinetics of IP administration [6]. A possible benefit of reducing the paclitaxel regimen to 3 h is a reduction of myelotoxicity. Metabolic and renal complications of cisplatin can be ameliorated by appropriate pre and posthydration and urinary output monitoring along with reducing the dose of IP cisplatin to 75 mg/m^2. Neurotoxicity may also be reduced by lowering the dose of cisplatin to 75 mg/m^2. Dose–response studies with cisplatin have not shown major differences in outcome in the 50–100 mg/m^2 range when cisplatin is given intravenously (IV). Toxicity may also be reduced by replacing cisplatin with carboplatin [2]. However, the efficacy of IP carboplatin has not been compared to IP cisplatin. The GOG initiated a series of phase I/II trials to establish experimental regimens for a new IP randomized clinical trial. Due to limitations of sample size and necessary accrual, the ideal five arm randomized trial is not feasible, and three arms had to be chosen.

Simultaneous with the work at GOG to improve the toxicity profile of IP chemotherapy, there has been documentation of the efficacy of bevacizumab in the treatment of recurrent ovarian cancer [8]. In August 2009, the three arm randomized clinical trial of primary treatment of ovarian cancer, with or without bevacizumab, concurrent with chemotherapy, and with and without consolidation, in addition to carboplatin and paclitaxel, GOG 0218, was completed [8, 9]. This study led to the application for FDA approval of bevacizumab for initial therapy with carboplatin plus paclitaxel in ovarian cancer. The Japanese GOG (JGOG) [10] has also demonstrated superiority (hazard ratio=0.72) of dose-dense weekly paclitaxel (80 mg/m^2, days 1, 8, and 15) and carboplatin (AUC=6, day 1), when compared to every 3 week paclitaxel (180 mg/m^2) and carboplatin (AUC=6). These advances in the treatment of primary ovarian cancer were incorporated into the GOG clinical trial, GOG 0252.

The three-arm randomized trial, GOG 0252, opened to accrual in July 2009. This study uses the results from GOG 0218 to test the addition of bevacizumab to IP chemotherapy with careful attention to toxicity as well as survival. It includes the JGOG IV dose-dense regimen of IV carboplatin (AUC=6, day 1), IV paclitaxel (80 mg/m^2, days 1, 8, and 15) and IV bevacizumab (15 mg/kg, day 1, beginning on cycle two) as the control arm [10]. The study includes two IP experimental arms: the IP carboplatin arm has an identical dose and schedule to the IV control arm only with the carboplatin dose being administered IP (AUC=6, IP, day 1); and the IP cisplatin arm, which is similar to GOG 0172, but attempts to reduce neuropathy by lowering the cisplatin dose and including a 3-h paclitaxel infusion to allow for outpatient administration. This experimental arm includes IV paclitaxel

Table 6.1 GOG 0252, three-arm randomized trial treatment arms

Arm I: IV control regimen	Paclitaxel 80 mg/m² IV over 1 h on day 1, 8, and 15, plus carboplatin AUC 6 IV on day 1 every 3 weeks for six cycles and bevacizumab 15 mg/kg IV during chemotherapy cycles two to six followed by bevacizumab 15 mg/kg IV every 3 weeks cycles 7–22 after the completion of chemotherapy
Arm II: IP experimental regimen	Paclitaxel 80 mg/m² IV over 1 h on days 1, 8, and 15, plus carboplatin AUC 6 IP on day 1, every 3 weeks for six cycles and bevacizumab 15 mg/kg IV during chemotherapy cycles two to six followed by bevacizumab 15 mg/kg IV every 3 weeks cycles 7–22 after the completion of chemotherapy
Arm III: IP experimental regimen	Paclitaxel 135 mg/m² IV over 3 h on day 1, followed by cisplatin 75 mg/m/² IP on day 2, followed by paclitaxel 60 mg/m² IP on day 8 every 3 weeks for six cycles and bevacizumab 15 mg/kg IV during chemotherapy cycles two to six followed by bevacizumab 15 mg/kg IV every 3 weeks cycles 7–22 after the completion of chemotherapy

(135 mg/m² over 3 h, day 1), IP cisplatin (75 mg/m², day 2), IP paclitaxel (60 mg/m², day 8), and IV bevacizumab (15 mg/kg, day 1, beginning on cycle two) The details of the treatment regimens for GOG 0252 are presented in Table 6.1.

Myelotoxicity will be expected in arm I and II, since only about half the participants in the JGOG study completed the protocol-directed therapy and the actual delivered mean relative dose intensity of the dose-dense regimen was actually lower than the standard every 3 week regimen [10]. Grade 3/4 neutropenia occurred in 94% and thrombocytopenia in 44% of patients, resulting in dose delays and reductions. Even with these adjustments, the weekly paclitaxel delivered a survival benefit. This survival benefit was similar to the previous high dose IP arm of GOG 0172, where most patients failed to complete six cycles and still a survival advantage was obtained [11]. In GOG 0252, Arm III should be very well tolerated due to the dose reductions from GOG 0172, and could conceivably have a superior survival result if completion rates of 90% are achieved instead of the 42% completion rate seen in GOG 0172. The addition of bevacizumab is expected to be well tolerated based on a number of phase I trials and GOG 0218 [9], without evidence of concern for excessive bowel complications. This three-arm trial will determine whether the survival advantage of the IP route of administration of chemotherapy is important enough, in the era of targeted agents and weekly paclitaxel, to overcome the toxicity and challenges of IP administration of cisplatin. It will also deliver an answer to the question proposed by Fujiwara, as to whether IP carboplatin can be substituted for IP cisplatin, without compromising survival [2].

6.2
Background on IP Catheters

Retrospective studies have documented the complications associated with chemotherapy administration through intraperitoneal catheters [4, 12–26]. Davidson et al. [15] reported on the use of a polyurethane fenestrated catheter (Port-A-Cath®) in 227 patients receiving

IP chemotherapy at Memorial Sloan Kettering Cancer Center. They noted inflow obstruction in 8.8%, infection in 5.3%, and bowel perforation in 3.5%, for a total catheter complication rate of 17.6%. As a follow-up, Makhija et al. [18] reported the change in catheters from the polyurethane *Port-A-Cath®* system, to a *Bardport®* 14.3 Fr fenestrated silicone peritoneal catheter at their institution. Catheters were placed at laparotomy in 69.6% of cases, 19.5% at laparoscopy, and 10.9% were placed at a separate procedure. Of the 301 patients, 10% of patients had catheter-related complications and 93% completed all of the prescribed chemotherapy. The type of catheter-related complications included malfunction in 6.3% and infection in 3.7% of cases. Five patients required catheter repair or replacement to complete their treatment. The change in the type of catheter as well as the avoidance of placement at the time of bowel resection was believed to decrease their complications from as high as 17.6% to 10%. Overall, this was considered a dramatic improvement from the Davidson report, since there were no major bowel injuries, and the complications were easily managed, with minimal disruption of treatment.

Walker et al. [27] reviewed the reasons for the discontinuation of IP therapy by 119 of the 205 patients who were randomized to the IP chemotherapy arm of GOG 0172 for optimal stage III ovarian cancer. Catheter-related complications were the primary reason for 34% (40/119) of the patients who discontinued IP chemotherapy or 19.5% of those randomized to the IP arm. These failures were attributed to infection (10.2% of all patients randomized to IP therapy), inflow obstruction (5%), port access problems (4%), and leaking (2%). It should be noted that during this prospective randomized trial, all patients were optimally surgically resected to 1 cm or less at initial treatment for epithelial ovary or peritoneal cancer, and were receiving the same chemotherapy regimen. It is one of the few reports of IP cisplatin at 100 mg/m^2 day 2 and IP paclitaxel 60 mg/m^2 day 8. This trial was conducted at multiple institutions with hundreds of surgeons using various devices. Bowel resections were performed in 32.2% of all study participants. Only 34% of the 50 patients with left colon resection completed six cycles. Sixteen percent never received the first cycle and 52% received two or fewer cycles. Bowel resection was the only surgical risk factor found in the analysis associated with failure to complete or begin IP therapy. This failure to complete or begin IP therapy may be unrelated to the colon resection, but related instead to the reluctance of patients and physicians to be committed to IP therapy when the patient may have poor physical status, be at higher risk of complications, and have gastrointestinal and nutritional issues.

In 1990, the University of Oklahoma began using the Bardport® venous access device (9.6 French) with a single lumen silicone catheter for IP administration, and this experience was reported by Landrum in 2008 [4]. The port is the same as described above with catheters that come either preattached or attachable. The attachable catheter is preferred in cases with delayed insertion as it provides the surgeon with increased flexibility in choices for placement. In this report, 12% of cases discontinued IP therapy due to catheter problems [4]. The silicone catheter, either venous access or peritoneal, does not appear to adhere to the bowel or cause peritoneal adhesions as was reported with the polyurethane, fenestrated catheter in the Davidson et al. [15] report. Earlier studies implemented the original Tenckhoff peritoneal dialysis catheter for use with ovarian cancer chemotherapy [28, 29]. These fenestrated catheters were noted to encourage fibrous sheath formation and subsequently adhesions leading to bowel obstruction [14]. A Dacron cuff was also present to secure the catheter along the abdominal wall and prevent migration [15]. There have been reports of migration of the Dacron cuff into the peritoneal cavity and erosion of catheters and dacron into small bowel, rectum, and vagina [12, 14, 16, 23, 25]. Because of these concerns, investigators at Memorial and Oklahoma now utilize silicone catheters without Dacron cuffs [4, 13]. Use of a silicone fenestrated or venous catheter is expected to be associated with approximately a 10% catheter complication rate. Differences in outcomes between the fenestrated IP Bardport and the Powerport polyurethane 8 Fr venous access catheter were evaluated by Ivy et al. [17]. The fenestrated port was associated with a 12% and the venous system with a 17% catheter-related complication rate.

Abdominal pain is a frequently reported complaint during the administration of IP chemotherapy [5]. The mechanism is poorly understood, but in the absence of peritonitis or bowel injury, abdominal pain may be a result of stretching and distension of bowel-to-bowel adhesions with the infusion of 2 L of saline. Abdominal pain may also indicate that drug distribution is less than ideal and limited to collections of drug in small pockets between adhesions. In most studies, the toxicity related to abdominal pain has been low grade and resolved with nonopioid treatment [8, 30]; however, physicians and patients should be cognizant of this potential complication. Higher pain rates may exist for paclitaxel IP infusion, since pain was a dose-limiting toxicity with IP doses greater than 175 mg/m^2 in the phase I study [31]. In GOG 0172, pain was the primary factor for the discontinuation of treatment in four patients and a contributing factor in another 16 patients [27]. A reduction in the volume of chemotherapy given or rate of infusion may decrease symptoms of pain. Paclitaxel has also been associated with bowel complications when given via the IV route, so there may be more pain and adhesion formation associated IP administration of this particular chemotherapeutic agent [32, 33]. Eighteen cases have been identified in the literature in which gastrointestinal necrosis or bowel perforation has occurred subsequent to IV paclitaxel administration [32, 33]. The investigators hypothesized that paclitaxel may directly act on compromised gastrointestinal epithelium and induce mitotic arrest, reducing the reparative capacity of the tissue. These bowel complications have been noted to occur roughly 2 weeks after cycle one or two is given. Clinically, these patients present with fever, neutropenia, and abdominal pain. Although relatively few cases have been reported, the mortality of these patients approaches 50%.

IP chemotherapy after neoadjuvant chemotherapy has tremendous appeal due to the improvement in the patient's physical status, nutritional status, and thus possibly, fewer IP chemotherapy complications. However, the estimated overall 5-year survival rate of 30% for secondary cytoreduction leaves room for improvement [34, 35]. The Southwest Oncology Group (SWOG) attempted to improve survival with the addition of IP chemotherapy after three cycles of IV carboplatin and paclitaxel and optimal interval debulking [36]. Unfortunately, after enrolling 56 eligible patients, only 36 women underwent interval debulking, and then only 26 received subsequent IP chemotherapy and 18 completed the protocol-specified therapy. Only one had a catheter complication. The median overall survival was only 32 months [36], which was similar to the European Organization for Research and Treatment of Cancer (EORTC) study [35].

6.3
Peritoneal Catheter Placement at Primary Surgery for Presumed Ovarian Cancer

Surgical treatment of a patient with a potential diagnosis of ovarian cancer requires an extensive education about the potential diagnosis, treatment options, and intraoperative decision making required by the gynecologic oncologist. This consenting process ideally includes information on procedures necessary for optimal surgical resection, staging, and placement of chemotherapy delivery devices. The decision to place an IP catheter should usually be the default position, when the diagnosis is uncertain. It is less costly, more convenient, and less disruptive for a patient to have the IP catheter removed if the final pathology results deem it unnecessary, rather than have it placed at a subsequent operation, after it is determined to be desirable.

6.4
Radical Surgical Procedures

There is a survival advantage provided by a complete resection of all ovarian cancer at the time of primary surgical debulking. Controversy persists on whether it is the tumor behavior that allows for the resectability, or the surgeons skill and training in aggressive upper abdominal procedures, which provide the ultimate result. There are certainly women presenting to gynecologic oncologists who are too old, frail, or medically compromised to survive radical procedures. The feasibility of complete resection and the judgment as to when it is appropriate to perform ultra radical procedures remains under debate [34].

The analysis of GOG 0172, a prospective clinical trial comparing IV vs. IP chemotherapy, documented the current state of surgical procedures used to obtain optimal surgical resection in women with stage III disease [27]. The results show that to obtain optimal resection additional procedures include: hysterectomy in 80%; appendectomy in 35%; left colon or recto-sigmoid resection in 24.3%; right colon in 8%; colostomy in 4%; and small bowel resection in 7%. The patient-specific bowel resection rate was 32.2%. Diaphragm resection and splenectomy were uncommon at that time, but appear to be increasingly used by recently trained gynecologic oncologists.

Furthermore, an analysis of how additional procedures may affect the patient tolerance of IP chemotherapy was performed [27]. The understanding of cause and effect may allow for changes in practice patterns, which could prevent some of the adverse outcomes.

Adverse outcomes observed with the administration of IP chemotherapy include: infection of the port site; peritonitis; abscess; port access problems; leaking; abdominal pain; bowel complications; infusion of the drugs into the gastrointestinal tract manifested as diarrhea; or out of the vagina or bladder, manifested as incontinence.

In GOG 0172, completion of six cycles was not found to be superior in those patients in whom the IP port was placed at the time of debulking surgery vs. those who had placement delayed until after wound healing [36]. Of the sixteen (8%) out of 205 patients who never received their first cycle of IP chemotherapy, nine (4%) never had an IP catheter placed. The hazard of not placing an IP catheter at the time of primary surgery is that one of the overall barriers to receiving IP chemotherapy is simply the placement of the delivery device. The practice of placing it at the time of primary debulking is very important when one understands the inertia that causes many patients to never have the opportunity to receive this choice of therapy. The potential benefit of delayed placement is that the potential complications of surgical healing will not complicate the function of the IP catheter. The potential surgical complications include anastamotic leak, pelvic abscess, sepsis, and wound infections, all of which could cause catheter infections.

Of the surgical procedures, only the left colon and recto-sigmoid resection are correlated with failure to complete six cycles of IP therapy. Only 34% of patients who underwent these procedures completed all six cycles, and 16% never received any IP chemotherapy. The conclusion could be drawn that failure to place the IP catheter caused many to never receive IP therapy. Another conclusion could be that these patients were slow to recover from the radical surgery and they would not tolerate another procedure. Many surgeons prefer to place the port in an uncomplicated colon resection where gross fecal contamination did not occur, others continue to prefer delayed placement until resumption of oral intake and good functional status. Catheter infections and peritonitis are potential sequelae of the placement of a foreign body during a contaminated surgical case. Currently, individualization on a case by case basis is needed until more data are generated.

6.5
Choice of Device and Catheter

IP chemotherapy is not new. IP therapy has a long history of utilizing peritoneal dialysis technology to provide delivery of drugs to the peritoneal cavity. The mixing of radical surgery with a foreign body in the peritoneal cavity has led to many reports of poor results in the past. There are two favored approaches to these devices and catheters today [4, 6, 13, 18]. One is to utilize the venous access technology with a completely implanted access port attached to a silicone catheter. The Bardport® brand has two preferred devices. Bard port silicone peritoneal catheter 14.3 Fr (reorder number 0603006) without a cuff is the preferred catheter for IP therapy. The Bardport MRI Implanted Port (reorder number 0602680) attachable 9.6 Fr open ended single lumen silicone venous catheter and the Titanium Dome Implanted Port with attachable 9.6 Fr open ended single lumen venous catheter (reorder number 0602870) are also available.

The 14.3 Fr peritoneal catheters are attachable to a port and can be cut to the proper length at each end. The fenestrated tip should not be long enough to reach the vagina, bladder, or any anastamosis site, and the multiple fenestrations must all be within the peritoneal cavity. The catheter within the abdominal wall and attached to the port must be free of fenestrations. Caution should be taken to avoid incorrect placement of the catheter. Tailoring is necessary for each individual patient, their postoperative anatomy, the port site selection, and peritoneal insertion site selection. This catheter is large, firm, and will not kink as it is brought through the abdominal wall. It can be used to aspirate back ascites, and generally works well since it is made of silicone. It does not form the fibrinous sheaths which were notorious in the past from fenestrated catheters made of other materials. The lack of a Dacron cuff improves the ease of removal. This catheter can be removed easily in the office, and it does not become densely adherent to the bowel wall or peritoneal adhesions.

Alternatively, the use of the venous access device with a silicone catheter, which is large and firm enough to prevent kinking, may be used. The Bardport 9.6 Fr silicone catheter, attachable to an implanted port, has been successfully used for decades. The only decision that is required for the placement is where to place the port and the tip. The tip must be placed where it will not be entrapped by adhesions, since there is only one location for the IP infusion to exit. If placed in the location of the omentectomy (i.e., between the transverse colon and the anterior abdominal wall) it will likely get trapped between the adhesions that develop in that location. If the right colon was not resected, the right side overlying the small bowel tends to be the location that is ideal. Alternatively, if an ileocecal resection was required, the opposite side is chosen.

6.6
Technique for Placement at Laparotomy

The access port must be supported by bone and fascia to aid nursing staff in palpating the device and improve Huber needle insertion accuracy. A device that is hidden in fat and tilts when accessed will cause access failures and potentially catheter lacerations with the needle. Unfortunately, without the aid of blood return as found in venous ports, the tactile sensation of the Huber needle going through the diaphragm and hitting the metal back of the port may be the only indication of successful access. Only a few patients will have ascites draw back at the time of accessing the port. Adequate amounts of adipose and skin overlying the port to prevent erosion is also important, and there are women who are too thin for this location. Low profile devices or an alternative site needs to be considered, and some have described the inguinal ligament.

At the completion of the ovarian cancer debulking and staging procedure, and just prior to closing the incision, make a 3–4-cm incision over the lower costal margin, at the midclavicular line or toward the anterior axillary line, on the side where the catheter is to be placed. Consideration of the patient preference is ideal, when feasible. Avoiding locations which could interfere with patient's usual sleeping positions, and preventing irritation from clothing, such as bra support straps, may improve patient satisfaction.

The incision is carried down to the fascia using blunt and sharp dissection. A subcutaneous pocket superior to the incision is fashioned slightly larger than the diameter of the portal. Select an area several centimeters (ideally 10 cm) from the port site for peritoneal entrance site of the catheter. Select a subcutaneous tunnel from the port pocket to the site for entrance into the peritoneal cavity, far away from the midline incision to avoid it getting caught in closing suture. Draw the catheter using a tunneling device, or long tonsil clamp, through the subcutaneous tissue just above the fascia for approximately 10 cm, and then penetrate the abdominal wall into the peritoneal cavity.

Be certain that all fenestrations are in the peritoneal cavity and not in the abdominal wall tunnel. Cut the catheter to proper length at both ends to fit the patient anatomy.

Attach the catheter to the port as per manufacturer's instructions, and suture the port in place in four corners with permanent suture (i.e., 2–0 prolene) to the fascia overlying the thorax. The use of vicryl, or absorbable suture, could allow the port to become mobile and flip over preventing access with a needle. Be sure that the chemotherapy nurses will be able to feel the port and stabilize it on the chest wall for easy access with Huber needle in the future. In addition, ensure that the Huber needle does not have to go through the suture line in the wound to access the port; the port should lie superior to the incision and suture line. The Huber needle should be able to penetrate healthy sterilized skin to access the port, far away from suture line and steri-strips and other contamination risks.

After flushing the system with heparin, 100 U/mL, to determine that flow is not obstructed and no leaks exist, place the distal end of the catheter to the desired infusion site, with at least 10 cm of free catheter in the abdomen. Do not allow the catheter to be long enough to reach the bladder, vagina, rectum, or any anastamosis sites.

Close incisions and place a Huber needle transdermally into the portal if the catheter is going to be utilized within a few days of the postoperative period. Wait for a minimum of 24 h prior to treating a patient after any IP port placement to allow for the peritoneal sealing of catheter insertion site. After laparotomy, wait for the return of gastrointestinal function and resolution of ileus, as indicated by having a regular diet that is tolerated and normal bowel movement. This verifies that it is unlikely that the patient is suffering a postoperative infection or major complication which could be compounded by chemotherapy toxicities.

6.7
Prevention of Catheter Failures

Complications of IP chemotherapy are best described as: (1) related to the peritoneal access device; (2) the peritoneal infusion of chemotherapy agents and the discomfort of abdominal distention with 2 L of saline; or (3) related to the systemic side effects of chemotherapy. The various catheter complications experienced by patients enrolled to IP therapy are summarized in Table 6.2. Each of the reported complications will be addressed and technical aspects of the care of these patients discussed below.

The failure to place a peritoneal access device is best overcome by placing it at the time of the original laparotomy. Each ovarian cancer treatment center must build their capacity and technological expertise to care for this very challenging patient population. When that has not occurred, a common mistake by surgeons is to reenter the abdomen through the original vertical incision. This technique is often complicated by enterotomies and bowel adhesions secondary to previous radical resection. The procedure is often abandoned due to adhesions, when an alternative procedure technique may have been successful. Knowledge of the operative report and disease resected at the previous procedure, allows one to avoid likely sites of adhesions. The transverse colon is generally adherent to the anterior

Table 6.2 Catheter complications

	Davidson et al. [15] (n=227)	Waggoner et al. [26] (n=24)	Sakuragi et al. [41] (n=78)	Makhija et al. [18] (n=301)	Fujiwara et al. [2] (n=165)	Walker et al. [27] (n=205)	Total subjects (n=1,000)
Malfunction	20 (8.8%)	2 (8.3%)	5 (6.4%)	19 (6.3%)	8 (4.8%)	58 (28.3%)	112 (11.2%)
Infection	12 (5.3%)	1 (4.2%)	16 (20.5%)	11 (3.7%)	4 (2.4%)	21 (10.2%)	65 (6.5%)
Abdominal pain	0	1 (4.2%)	3 (3.8%)	0	3 (1.8%)	20/119 (16.8%)	27 (2.7%)
Bowel perforation	8 (3.5%)	0	1 (1.2%)	0	0	4 (2%)	13 (1.3%)
SBO/Ileus	0	0	1 (1.2%)	0	1 (0.6%)	0	2 (0.2%)

abdominal wall due to the omentectomy. Utilization of the left upper quadrant access via laparoscopy or right lower quadrant infraumbilical site over the cecum for mini-laparotomy, can be alternatives, depending on previous surgical procedures [4, 6, 11, 37].

There have been cases in which the IP catheter and access port were placed but never functioned. To avoid this, it is important to be sure the IP port is functional prior to leaving the operating room initially. Good flow with saline throughout the procedure is important to document, since the catheter can be kinked with the closing sutures. Documentation of function in the surgical setting is helpful. The last step is the infusion of heparin 100 U/cm^3 to be sure of good flow and maintain patency after all incisions are closed.

When malfunction is identified in the chemotherapy suite, fluoroscopy can be utilized to be sure that the Huber needle is in the reservoir and watch the contrast as it goes into the catheter. Problems can include kinking of the tubing, adhesions around the outflow tract of the catheter, disconnection of the tubing from the reservoir, and migration of the catheter backward into the port pocket. When the outflow of the catheter is obstructed by adhesions, the fluid infused into the port will track back along the side of the catheter and into the port pocket. Surgical interventions can be planned based on the results of the fluoroscopy.

Secondary inflow obstruction in a previously functioning catheter may be due to a peritoneal reaction to the catheter or the chemotherapy causing adhesions surrounding and obstructing inflow. Fluoroscopy is helpful to decide whether surgical correction should be considered.

The inability to gain access to the port reservoir can be due to poor site selection, obesity, or the flipping over of the port so that the diaphragm is no longer available. These problems can be prevented and corrected.

The selection of a firm platform for the port to be sutured allows for easy palpation of the dome or diaphragm of the reservoir, except in the case of morbid obesity. The sutures need to be permanent 2–0 prolene to prevent tilt or inversion of the port. This allows the oncology nursing staff to feel the port and direct the needle into the reservoir until they feel the metal back of the device. This will indicate that the needle is long enough to infuse. Improper choice of needle length and poor positioning of the patient are very simple mistakes that can be overcome. The needle must be long enough to hit the metal plate on the far side of the diaphragm, or the needle is at risk of being dislodged and infusing the chemotherapy into the subcutaneous tissues. The availability of beds in the chemotherapy suite has been a deficiency in the past, but the supine position is ideal for IP port access and to prevent dislodging of needles during infusion secondary to movement. Always remove steri-strips from the wounds and perform proper cleaning of the healthy skin overlying the port with betadine or chloroprep. There should not be an incision immediately overlying the port diagram or there may be increased infection rates or pain. Some surgeons chose to make the port pocket incision cephalad to the port in order to better displace the incision site from the port needle insertion site.

Port leakage can occur into the subcutaneous tissues, out of the port wound, the midline wound, the vagina, bladder, or rectum. Patients' complaints of urinary incontinence or diarrhea need to be investigated as a potential IP catheter complication. Each problem may have a separate cause, and again fluoroscopy can be very helpful. Leaking out of the port wound can be due to a failure to get the Huber needle into the reservoir. The needle could have lacerated the catheter, causing leakage into the tissues, or the catheter could dislodge from the port. Most commonly, it appears that the fluid goes down the catheter, and then due to obstruction in the peritoneal cavity, tracks back around the catheter into the port pocket.

Removal of the IP port along with its catheter, as a minor bedside procedure, is usually all that is required to correct the vaginal, bladder, or bowel fistula. Patients tend to heal spontaneously, and no laparotomy is required. Foley catheter drainage is recommended in the case of a bladder perforation. Observation of the patient for fever, peritonitis, and elevated neutrophils is appropriate for bowel injury. Most reports indicate spontaneous closure as the most common outcome. Continuing with IV chemotherapy when the patient has recovered is recommended in these situations.

For the prevention of fistulas, careful attention to vaginal cuff closure, supracervical hysterectomy, and avoidance of too lengthy a catheter are recommended. The migration of the catheter into the bladder or bowel would likely involve the catheter to be long enough to reach an injured structure to which it became attached by adhesions. In addition, prevention requires careful attention to the site selection for the ports and catheters which are tailored to patients postoperative surgical weaknesses. The most important prevention strategy is to remove an IP port and catheter as soon as it is not being utilized, since it can only cause harm.

Infection of the port pocket may be an immediate postoperative complication, or a result of a subsequent cellulitis or peritonitis. Many patients have subclinical low-grade infections or poorly healing wounds after a major debulking surgery. Infection, seroma, or dehiscence of the primary midline incision will certainly contribute to an increased risk of port site infections. Delay of chemotherapy until the wound is well healed is ideal, but not always feasible. Competing risks must be prioritized. Wound vacuum-assisted closure (VAC) has improved the speed of healing and appears to isolate the actively healing wound from the port incision.

Subclinical intraabdominal or pelvic abscesses may become evident with IP chemotherapy. Poorly healing bowel anastamosis sites may leak after IP chemotherapy (and possibly be accentuated by paclitaxel). Awareness of the possibility of these events will improve the speed of interventions. Patients who are failing to recover from their surgery need investigation to determine if low-grade fevers or elevated neutrophils are indicating that a computerized tomography (CT) scan may be warranted to search for abscesses or leaks. Resumption of appetite and regular dietary intake will generally indicate that the patient is ready for chemotherapy administration.

The suspicion of peritonitis following chemotherapy can be investigated by the aspiration of peritoneal fluid from the IP port site. Gram stain and culture can be helpful to make a rapid diagnosis and direct appropriate treatment. Removal of IP ports and catheters once infection has been documented, including a treatment delay for resumption using the IV route, is preferred.

Bowel obstruction, perforation, or fistula may be unrelated or a direct result of IP chemotherapy. These events are too infrequent to generalize as to the cause, but speculation is possible. Surgical intervention after IP chemotherapy usually identifies peritoneal thickening, pseudo capsules, and adhesions that appear to be a peritoneal reaction to the chemotherapy agents. This can make repair of the problem more challenging. Avoiding laparotomy, when the only intervention that may be necessary is the removal of the Port and catheter, and intravenous antibiotics should be considered. CT scan results will guide decision making.

Pain during infusion could be secondary to the large volume (2,000 cm³) of saline for dilution, pulling and distorting bowel adhesions, or a direct toxicity of the drug. Infusion of the initial bolus of chemotherapy in a smaller volume and then added additional saline allows for the full dose of drug to be delivered, even if the patient will not tolerate a full 2 L of fluid. In general, pain will not persist beyond a few hours of the treatment upon resorption of the fluid. There may be a patient-specific paclitaxel-derived abdominal pain response. This could be an allergic-type response or vesicant-like reaction to the drug. Most paclitaxel extravasations from failed venous infusions result in some skin discoloration and inflammation without necrosis. A new IP port on the opposite side of the abdomen may be successful at resuming IP chemotherapy. Unfortunately, abdominal pain requiring narcotics and discontinuation of infusion have a low likelihood of being corrected, and intravenous infusion should be considered.

6.8
Prevention of Adhesions

Many adhesion prevention strategies are commercially available. Seprafilm®, a sodium hyaluronate-carboxymethylcellulose (HA-CMC) barrier, is most widely marketed for the prevention of adhesions of the anterior abdominal wall to the underlying bowel. A randomized trial of patients undergoing colorectal surgery with a laparoscopic observation of adhesion outcome has demonstrated efficacy for this purpose [38]. It is thought that Seprafilm application will improve the distribution of IP chemotherapy by preventing peritoneal adhesions, since it has been shown to decrease adhesions at the time of ovarian cancer cytoreduction [39]. There is concern about increased loculated fluid collections and possibly increased infection and bowel obstructions following Seprafilm application [40]. It may be possible to avoid intervention for these finding on CT scan if the patient appears well, as they are likely to resolve without complication [8].

6.9
Delayed Insertion of Peritoneal Catheter

Surgical implantation with mini-laparotomy procedures viewable on video is available at the Society of Gynecologic Oncologists (sgo.org) and GOG (gog.org) websites. There are several key points for delayed insertion procedures that can reduce future complications:

1. Do not use the previous midline incision for delayed IP port placement. Select a site several centimeters below and lateral to the umbilicus (often overlying the cecum) and make an incision through the skin, subcutaneous tissue, and fascia. Separate the rectus muscle and enter the peritoneum. Knowledge of the previous surgical resections and

current anatomy will assist in choosing a location which is less likely to have anterior abdominal wall adhesions. The transverse colon will be adherent to the anterior abdominal wall from the previous omentectomy. The vertical midline incision will have small bowel adhesions.

2. Pull the catheter from the subcutaneous tissue into the peritoneal cavity through the full thickness of the abdominal wall (fascia, muscle, peritoneum) from an adjacent location (not through the incision) while under direct visualization to prevent injury to the bowel. This can be accomplished with a tonsil clamp or tunneling device. Closing the minilap incision around the catheter may allow for leakage through the wound and migration of the catheter into the abdominal wall.

3. The catheter must be left in the abdominal cavity at least 10 cm to prevent migration out of the peritoneal cavity.

4. The opposite end of the catheter is tunneled up to the costal margin where it is attached to an implanted port as described above.

5. The catheter is left long enough to not retract, but not long enough to reach any bowel anastamosis site, or the vagina, rectum, or bladder. It is generally left at least 10 cm into the peritoneal cavity.

Recommendations for surgical implantation using laparoscopy include [11]:

1. Laparoscopic placement of an IP catheter is usually feasible from a left upper quadrant approach. Knowledge of the previous procedures performed (i.e., bowel resections and reanastamosis sites) and previous location of the tumor will inform the surgeon as to the best approach and the locations to avoid.

2. Once the peritoneal cavity can be visualized, a second puncture can be used to gain access to the peritoneal cavity for the catheter, and then the catheter tunneled in the subcutaneous tissues to the planned Port pocket. Closure of the peritoneal and fascia port sites with a Carter Thompson suture passing device may help avoid leaking, as long as the catheter is not lacerated or kinked.

3. Trochar site tumor implantation is a concern surrounding this technique [41]. The rapid administration of chemotherapy after laparoscopy is the likely solution to this problem.

6.10
Interventional Radiology Placement

Interventional radiology may place IP ports in some institutions [42, 43]. This requires effective communication between the surgeon and the radiologist for optimal results. Knowledge of the anatomy and best sites for peritoneal access should be communicated. The presence of ascites greatly facilitates catheter placement. CT or ultrasound-directed access to the peritoneal cavity can allow catheter placement and then subcutaneous tunneling of the catheter to the lower chest wall for appropriate subcutaneous port placement and catheter attachment.

6.11
Removal of the Catheter

Removal of the IP port and catheter is performed as an office procedure with local anesthetic. The most difficult part of the procedure is getting into the pseudocapsule surrounding the port and the catheter. The next challenge is identification and removal of all four prolene sutures. The catheter slides out of the peritoneal cavity without difficulty. The port pocket is then closed in two layers. It is advised to remove the catheter as soon as it is no longer needed. Late complications can occur when the device is not being used [25].

6.12
Conclusions

Jaaback and colleagues completed a meta-analysis of clinical trials from 1,819 patients, documenting an overall survival benefit related to IP therapy (hazard ratio = 0.80) [30]. However, the expected toxicities must be understood and adequately managed. The National Cancer Institute released a Clinical Announcement in January 2006 summarizing for clinicians and the public the evidence required for their "strong consideration" of the use of intraperitoneal cisplatin chemotherapy for optimally resected stage III ovarian cancer patients [44].

The appropriate patient selection for IP chemotherapy had previously been limited to optimally resected stage III patients, but others have been seriously considered (i.e., stage II). GOG Protocol 0252 allows the enrollment of Stages II-IV. Select patients with early stage disease may benefit from this treatment route; however, there is concern that many patients with early disease are unlikely to recur and should not be subjected to the potential toxicity of IP cisplatin. Patients with suboptimal disease have also been considered to potentially benefit from IP therapy; however, the median survival of these patients is approximately 3 years, and the palliation of symptoms and quality of life outcomes may be the most appropriate measures of treatment benefit. There is also consideration of using IP therapy in patients with stage IV disease based only on a pleural effusion and without CT scan evidence of disease outside of the peritoneal cavity.

The choice of drugs, route, and schedule continues to need refinement to deliver the most efficacious results encompassing survival, quality of life, and toxicity. GOG 0252 (discussed above) is a clinical trial attempting to complete that task. The importance of a liter of normal saline intravenous prehydration prior to IP cisplatin and repeated after IP administration cannot be overemphasized. The development of the antiemetic guidelines by the American Society of Clinical Oncology (ASCO) [3] and the National Comprehensive Cancer Network (NCCN) [45] for the support of patients receiving cisplatin, should help all the patients to receive pretreatment with corticosteroids, $5-HT_3$ serotonin receptor inhibitor, and 1-NK receptor antagonist (aprepitant). These advances should help keep patients hydrated, nourished, and improve tolerance of this intense regimen.

References

1. Armstrong DK, Bundy B, Wenzel L, Huang HQ, Baergen R, Lele S et al (2006) Intraperitoneal cisplatin and paclitaxel in ovarian cancer. N Engl J Med 354(1):34–43
2. Fujiwara K, Sakuragi N, Suzuki S, Yoshida N, Maehata K, Nishiya M et al (2003) First-line intraperitoneal carboplatin-based chemotherapy for 165 patients with epithelial ovarian carcinoma: results of long-term follow-up. Gynecol Oncol 90(3):637–643
3. Kris MG, Hesketh PJ, Somerfield MR, Feyer P, Clark-Snow R, Koeller JM et al (2006) American Society of Clinical Oncology guideline for antiemetics in oncology: update 2006. J Clin Oncol 24(18):2932–2947
4. Landrum LM, Gold MA, Moore KN, Myers TK, McMeekin DS, Walker JL (2008) Intraperitoneal chemotherapy for patients with advanced epithelial ovarian cancer: a review of complications and completion rates. Gynecol Oncol 108(2):342–347
5. Wenzel LB, Huang HQ, Armstrong DK, Walker JL, Cella D (2007) Health-related quality of life during and after intraperitoneal versus intravenous chemotherapy for optimally debulked ovarian cancer: a Gynecologic Oncology Group Study. J Clin Oncol 25(4):437–443
6. Markman M, Walker JL (2006) Intraperitoneal chemotherapy of ovarian cancer: a review, with a focus on practical aspects of treatment. J Clin Oncol 24(6):988–994
7. Ozols RF, Bundy BN, Greer BE, Fowler JM, Clarke-Pearson D, Burger RA et al (2003) Phase III trial of carboplatin and paclitaxel compared with cisplatin and paclitaxel in patients with optimally resected stage III ovarian cancer: a Gynecologic Oncology Group study. J Clin Oncol 21(17):3194–3200
8. Burger RA, Sill MW, Monk BJ, Greer BE, Sorosky JI (2007) Phase II trial of bevacizumab in persistent or recurrent epithelial ovarian cancer or primary peritoneal cancer: a Gynecologic Oncology Group Study. J Clin Oncol 25(33):5165–5171
9. Burger RA, Brady M, Bookman MA et al (2010) Phase III trial of bevacizumab (BEV) in the primary treatment of advanced epithelial ovarian cancer (EOC), primary peritoneal cancer (PPC) or fallopian tube cancer (FTC): Gynecologic Oncology Group Study 218. ASCO. Abstract 52788
10. Katsumata N, Yasuda M, Takahashi F, Isonishi S, Jobo T, Aoki D et al (2009) Dose-dense paclitaxel once a week in combination with carboplatin every 3 weeks for advanced ovarian cancer: a phase 3, open-label, randomised controlled trial. Lancet 374(9698):1331–1338
11. Anaf V, Gangji D, Simon P, Saylam K (2003) Laparoscopical insertion of intraperitoneal catheters for intraperitoneal chemotherapy. Acta Obstet Gynecol Scand 82(12):1140–1145
12. Bilsel Y, Balik E, Bugra D, Yamaner S, Akyuz A (2005) A case of protrusion of an intraperitoneal chemotherapy catheter through rectum. Int J Gynecol Cancer 15(1):171–174
13. Black D, Levine DA, Nicoll L, Chou JF, Iasonos A, Brown CL et al (2008) Low risk of complications associated with the fenestrated peritoneal catheter used for intraperitoneal chemotherapy in ovarian cancer. Gynecol Oncol 109(1):39–42
14. Braly P, Doroshow J, Hoff S (1986) Technical aspects of intraperitoneal chemotherapy in abdominal carcinomatosis. Gynecol Oncol 25(3):319–333
15. Davidson SA, Rubin SC, Markman M, Jones WB, Hakes TB, Reichman B et al (1991) Intraperitoneal chemotherapy: analysis of complications with an implanted subcutaneous port and catheter system. Gynecol Oncol 41(2):101–106
16. Ghosh K, Geller MA, Twiggs LB (2000) Erosion of an intraperitoneal chemotherapy catheter resulting in an enterovaginal fistula. Gynecol Oncol 77(2):327–329
17. Ivy JJ, Geller M, Pierson SM, Jonson AL, Argenta PA (2009) Outcomes associated with different intraperitoneal chemotherapy delivery systems in advanced ovarian carcinoma: a single institution's experience. Gynecol Oncol 114(3):420–423

18. Makhija S, Leitao M, Sabbatini P, Bellin N, Almadrones L, Leon L et al (2001) Complications associated with intraperitoneal chemotherapy catheters. Gynecol Oncol 81(1):77–81
19. Pfeiffer P, Asmussen L, Kvist-Poulsen H, Bertelsen K (1989) Intraperitoneal chemotherapy: introduction of a new "single use" delivery system–a preliminary report. Gynecol Oncol 35(1):47–49
20. Pfeifle CE, Howell SB, Markman M, Lucas WE (1984) Totally implantable system for peritoneal access. J Clin Oncol 2(11):1277–1280
21. Piccart MJ, Speyer JL, Markman M, ten Bokkel Huinink WW, Alberts D, Jenkins J et al (1985) Intraperitoneal chemotherapy: technical experience at five institutions. Semi Oncol 12(3 suppl 4):90–96
22. Rubin SC, Hoskins WJ, Markman M, Hakes T, Lewis JL Jr (1989) Long-term access to the peritoneal cavity in ovarian cancer patients. Gynecol Oncol 33(1):46–48
23. Runowicz CD, Dottino PR, Shafir MK, Mark MA, Cohen CJ (1986) Catheter complications associated with intraperitoneal chemotherapy. Gynecol Oncol 24(1):41–50
24. van Dam PA, DeCloedt J, Tjalma WA, Buytaert P, Becquart D, Vergote IB (1999) Trocar implantation metastasis after laparoscopy in patients with advanced ovarian cancer: can the risk be reduced? Am J Obstet Gynecol 181(3):536–541
25. Varney RR, Goel R, vanSonnenberg E, Lucas WE, Casola G (1989) Delayed erosion of intraperitoneal chemotherapy catheters into the bowel. Report of two cases. Cancer 64(3):762–764
26. Waggoner SE, Johnson J, Barter J, Barnes W (1994) Intraperitoneal therapy administered through a Groshong catheter. Gynecol Oncol 53(3):320–325
27. Walker JL, Armstrong DK, Huang HQ, Fowler J, Webster K, Burger RA et al (2006) Intraperitoneal catheter outcomes in a phase III trial of intravenous versus intraperitoneal chemotherapy in optimal stage III ovarian and primary peritoneal cancer: a Gynecologic Oncology Group Study. Gynecol Oncol 100(1):27–32
28. Tenckhoff H, Schechter H (1968) A bacteriologically safe peritoneal access device. Trans Am Soc Artif Intern Organs 14:181–187
29. Wilkins ES (1991) Tissue reaction to intraperitoneally implanted catheter materials. J Biomed Eng 13(2):173–175
30. Jaaback K, Johnson N (2006) Intraperitoneal chemotherapy for the initial management of primary epithelial ovarian cancer. Cochrane database of systematic reviews (Online). (1):CD005340
31. Markman M, Rowinsky E, Hakes T, Reichman B, Jones W, Lewis JL Jr et al (1992) Phase I trial of intraperitoneal taxol: a Gynecoloic Oncology Group study. J Clin Oncol 10(9):1485–1491
32. Rose PG, Piver MS (1995) Intestinal perforation secondary to paclitaxel. Gynecol Oncol 57(2):270–272
33. Seewaldt VL, Cain JM, Goff BA, Tamimi H, Greer B, Figge D (1997) A retrospective review of paclitaxel-associated gastrointestinal necrosis in patients with epithelial ovarian cancer. Gynecol Oncol 67(2):137–140
34. Vergote I, Trope C, Amant F et al (2010) Neoadjuvant chemotherapy or primary surgery in stage IIIC-IV ovarian cancer. NEJM in press
35. Vergote I, De Wever I, Tjalma W, Van Gramberen M, Decloedt J, van Dam P (1998) Neoadjuvant chemotherapy or primary debulking surgery in advanced ovarian carcinoma: a retrospective analysis of 285 patients. Gynecol Oncol 71(3):431–436
36. Tiersten AD, Liu PY, Smith HO, Wilczynski SP, Robinson WR 3rd, Markman M et al (2009) Phase II evaluation of neoadjuvant chemotherapy and debulking followed by intraperitoneal chemotherapy in women with stage III and IV epithelial ovarian, fallopian tube or primary peritoneal cancer: Southwest Oncology Group Study S0009. Gynecol Oncol 112(3):444–449
37. Arts HJ, Willemse PH, Tinga DJ, de Vries EG, van der Zee AG (1998) Laparoscopic placement of PAP catheters for intraperitoneal chemotherapy in ovarian carcinoma. Gynecol Oncol 69(1):32–35

38. Becker JM, Stucchi AF (2004) Intra-abdominal adhesion prevention: are we getting any closer? Ann Surg 240(2):202–204
39. Bristow RE, Montz FJ (2005) Prevention of adhesion formation after radical oophorectomy using a sodium hyaluronate-carboxymethylcellulose (HA-CMC) barrier. Gynecol Oncol 99(2):301–308
40. Leitao MM Jr, Natenzon A, Abu-Rustum NR, Chi DS, Sonoda Y, Levine DA et al (2009) Postoperative intra-abdominal collections using a sodium hyaluronate-carboxymethylcellu-lose (HA-CMC) barrier at the time of laparotomy for ovarian, fallopian tube, or primary peritoneal cancers. Gynecol Oncol 115(2):204–208
41. Sakuragi N, Nakajima A, Nomura E, Noro N, Yamada H, Yamamoto R et al (2000) Complications relating to intraperitoneal administration of cisplatin or carboplatin for ovarian carcinoma. Gynecol Oncol 79(3):420–423
42. Orsi F, Della Vigna P, Penco S, Bonomo G, Lovati E, Bellomi M (2004) Percutaneous placement of peritoneal port-catheter in oncologic patients. Eur Radiol 14(11):2020–2024
43. Rundback JH, Gray RJ, Buck DR, Dolmatch BL, Haffner GH, Horton KM et al (1994) Fluoroscopically guided peritoneal catheter placement for intraperitoneal chemotherapy. J Vasc Interv Radiol 5(1):161–165
44. Trimble EL, Alvarez RD (2006) Intraperitoneal chemotherapy and the NCI clinical announcement. Gynecol Oncol 103(2 suppl 1):S18–S19
45. Ettinger DS, Armstrong DK, Barbour S, Berger MJ, Bierman PJ, Bradbury B et al (2009) Antiemesis. Clinical Practice Guidelines in Oncology. J Natl Compr Canc Netw 7(5):572–595

Selection of Drugs for Intraperitoneal Chemotherapy for Ovarian Cancer

7

Stephen B. Howell

7.1
Introduction

One of the characteristic features of ovarian cancer is that malignant cells shed from the primary tumor establish metastases that grow on the surface of the peritoneum. As these nodules expand, they derive a blood supply from peritoneal vessels, but tend not to invade through the peritoneal surface until later in the disease process. Because these nodules have a free surface in the peritoneal cavity and many types of drugs can be placed directly in this cavity, there is the opportunity to deliver chemotherapeutic agents at high concentration right to the surface of the tumor when the drugs are administered intraperitoneally. The hypothesis upon which the practice of intraperitoneal (IP) chemotherapy is based is that IP administration will increase the total drug exposure for the tumor over and above that which can be attained when a maximum tolerated dose of the same drug or drug combination is administered by the intravenous (IV) route. This chapter reviews the basic pharmacologic principles that provide guidance for the selection of drugs optimally used by the IP route and identifies the limitations and future promise of this mode of treatment.

IP chemotherapy clearly increases the survival of the subset of ovarian cancer patients who have small volume disease; this has now been demonstrated in multiple randomized trials [1]. Thus the basic pharmacologic principles of IP therapy that were first enunciated by Dedrick et al. [2] have been validated in patients. However, these trials have also established that the magnitude of the improvement in progression-free and overall survival is not large and that this route of administration is accompanied by adverse events not encountered with IV administration of the same drugs. Thus strategies for further improving the efficacy of IP therapy are being actively sought.

The concept upon which IP chemotherapy is based is that administration of a drug by the IP route allows one to deliver more drug exposure to the tumor without increasing the amount of drug reaching dose-limiting normal tissues. When tested against cultured tumor cell lines,

S.B. Howell
Department of Medicine and the Moores Cancer Center,
University of California, 3855 Health Sciences Drive,
La Jolla, CA, 92093-0819, USA
e-mail: showell@ucsd.edu

D.S. Alberts et al. (eds.), *Intraperitoneal Therapy for Ovarian Cancer*,
DOI: 10.1007/978-3-642-12130-2_7, © Springer-Verlag Berlin Heidelberg 2010

cytotoxic drugs reliably produce greater cell kill as total drug exposure is increased; the higher the drug concentration and the longer the duration of exposure, the greater the fraction of cells killed. The situation is more complex in vivo because of the greater heterogeneity of individual cells and surrounding environment. Increases in drug exposure do not always result in a proportional increase in tumor response. Some tumor cells reside close to a capillary and their exposure may vary directly with changes in the area under the plasma concentration time curve (AUC). However, cells that reside in hypoxic areas far from a capillary may have proportionally a much smaller increase in drug exposure for a given increase in plasma AUC. In addition, there is likely to be greater heterogeneity in the intrinsic resistance of tumor cells to drugs in vivo than in vitro. Tumor stem cells appear to express defense mechanisms that render them substantially more resistant than their more differentiated daughters, and the in vivo environment may heighten this disparity. Nonetheless, large increases in the amount of drug delivered to the tumor do generally result in greater tumor responses in murine tumor models and in patients. However, when drugs are given by the IV route, the doses needed to result in sufficient tumor cell killing to be detectable as a change in tumor volume are often substantially greater than can be tolerated by the normal tissues of the body.

7.2
Pharmacologic Principles of Intraperitoneal Therapy

The pharmacology of drugs injected into the peritoneal cavity is generally well-described by a two-compartment model in which one compartment is the cavity in which the tumor resides and the other is the blood compartment and all the other organs of the body. The total drug exposure for the peritoneal cavity and plasma is determined by measuring the concentration of drug in each compartment as a function of time after injection and integrating the area under the concentration-time curve (AUC). The relative advantage of giving a drug by the IP route can be expressed as the ratio of the AUC for the peritoneal cavity to that for the plasma. If the IP dose is large enough so that the plasma AUC due to drug leaking into the systemic circulation is as large as can be tolerated, drug delivery to the tumor via capillary flow will not be compromised and the tumor is expected to receive an additional increment of drug due to diffusion into the nodules from their free surface in the peritoneal cavity (free surface diffusion).

7.3
Relative Clearances and First Pass Metabolism

After injection into the peritoneal cavity, drugs can undergo inactivating metabolism in the cavity or leak into the systemic circulation through absorption into visceral or parietal peritoneal capillaries or the rich lymphatic network in the diaphragm that drains the cavity. None of the drugs most commonly used for IP chemotherapy undergo much metabolism in the peritoneal cavity itself. The rate at which their concentration in the cavity drops is a function of the surface area available for diffusion, the permeability of this surface, the volume of drug-containing fluid, and the difference in free drug concentration between the cavity and the plasma. Under steady-state conditions, the cavity-to-plasma concentration ratio is given by the following equation:

$$\frac{C_{\text{peritoneum}}}{C_{\text{plasma}}} = \frac{(\text{plasma clearance}) + (\text{cavity clearance})}{(\text{cavity clearance})} \tag{7.1}$$

This equation indicates that anything that increases the plasma clearance or decreases clearance from the cavity will increase the concentration ratio. Since AUC is determined by concentration times time, this equation also predicts the cavity-to-plasma concentration ratio. The ideal drug for IP chemotherapy would be one that has a very hard time getting out of the peritoneal cavity but that is cleared very rapidly once it reaches the plasma. This would result in a situation in which the peritoneal cavity concentration would remain high for a long period of time, but where there would be little opportunity for drug reaching the plasma to reach levels that are damaging for dose-limiting for normal tissues, such as the bone marrow or gut mucosa. Drugs that are large (e.g., high molecular weight), charged, or not very lipid soluble generally have a difficult time crossing lipid membranes and are expected to have low peritoneal clearances. However, the AUC ratio is determined by both the peritoneal and the plasma clearances and these characteristics also affect the plasma clearance. Therefore, the relative advantage of IP administration cannot be predicted based on these features alone. Nevertheless, Eq. (7.1) provides reasonable estimates of the relative advantage of administering a drug by the IP route.

The actual route of absorption of a drug from the peritoneal cavity also affects the AUC ratio since this can determine how much of the drug is inactivated by metabolism during transit. If the drug is inactivated during transit, the net effect is the same as increasing the plasma clearance. Drugs in the molecular weight range of the commonly used chemotherapeutic agents are absorbed primarily into the portal circulation that drains the visceral peritoneum, omentum, and mesentery, which together account for most of the surface area to which intraperitoneally instilled drugs have access. The parietal peritoneum is the only surface that drains directly into the systemic circulation. There is a rich network of lymphatics on the undersurface of the diaphragm that plays an important role in the removal of high molecular weight compounds from the peritoneal cavity; however, for small drugs with molecular weights less than 1,000 Da, this route contributes relatively little to the clearance in part because the flow rate in the lymphatics is so much less than in the portal circulation. Since low molecular weight drugs exit the peritoneal cavity primarily via the portal circulation, if they undergo extensive first pass metabolism in the liver, the amount of active drug reaching the systemic circulation per unit time can be quite small. Thus drugs such as cytarabine, 5-fluorouracil, 6-thioguanine, and floxuridine have AUC ratios that far exceed those of drugs with little hepatic first pass metabolism such as cisplatin and carboplatin.

7.4
Tumor Penetration

In order to be effective in reducing tumor burden in patients with ovarian cancer, an intraperitoneally instilled drug must penetrate into tumor nodules as well as enter cells that are floating free in the cavity. In spite of the fact that very high concentrations of drug may be present at the surface of a nodule growing on the peritoneal surface, there are a number of obstacles that limit penetration beyond the first few millimeters. First, as the drug enters cells in the outermost layers, there are fewer molecules left to diffuse to the next deeper layer. Second, tumor capillaries act like a sink drawing drug out of the nodule. Tumor capillaries are hyperpermeable, so that drug diffusing through the tumor interstitium can enter them easily. Given that the concentration of the drug in the blood is generally much lower than in the peritoneum, there is a substantial concentration gradient driving drug into the capillary. Capillary area and permeability, blood flow, and the diffusion coefficient of the drug in the tumor are key determinants of the extent to which blood flow in tumor capillaries limits free surface diffusion [3]. Third, the drug may be inactivated as it diffuses in from the surface of the nodule by binding to proteins in the extracellular matrix or by metabolism. Finally, tumor nodules typically have poorly formed or nonfunctional lymphatics and interstitial fluid moves from the interior of a nodule toward the edge. Thus a drug diffusing into a nodule from the surface must move upstream against a convective flow. As shown schematically in Fig. 7.1, all of these factors result in a concentration gradient of drug that decreases as one moves from the surface to the interior of the tumor nodule.

These considerations yield several predictions. First, since diffusion coefficients of the drugs that are used for IP chemotherapy are generally low, tumor volume can be expected to be a major determinant of the increase in drug exposure for the tumor attainable with IP instillation. Second, the depth at which cytotoxic concentrations of drug diffusing from the surface can be attained will be greater for poorly vascularized than for well-vascularized nodules. Finally, the peritoneal-to-plasma AUC ratio will exceed the tumor nodule to plasma AUC ratio. There is a large amount of variation between both patients and individual tumor nodules in the factors that determine depth of penetration. The interaction of these factors results in some predictions that may seem counterintuitive. For example, one would predict that drug penetration would be better: (1) in poorly vascularized nodules; (2) for large drugs that have difficulty getting into capillaries and thus will not be swept out of

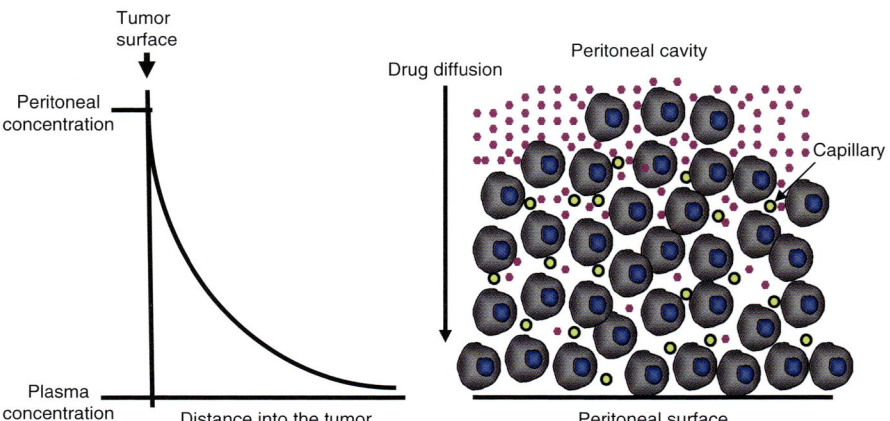

Fig. 7.1 Schematic diagram of the decrease in drug concentration as a function of distance of penetration into a tumor nodule. Redrawn from Dedrick and Flessner [3]

the nodule as readily; (3) nonreactive drugs that do not bind extensively to extracellular matrix; (4) drugs that are not rapidly transported into tumor cells; and (5) drugs that are not metabolized to inactive forms either in the extracellular matrix or inside tumor cells.

The importance of the ability of capillaries to limit drug penetration is exemplified by the gut. The crypt cells of the intestinal epithelium are rarely more than 1 mm from the visceral peritoneum and thus one might expect them to be at risk for damage as a result of the very high drug concentrations in the peritoneal cavity. However, IP chemotherapy rarely produces damage to the gut epithelium even under circumstances where the drug doses are high enough to cause other types of adverse events. This is likely due to the existence of a very extensive and high flow rate capillary network in the submucosa that functions to intercept drug diffusing through the visceral peritoneum and sweep it into the bloodstream.

Clinical trials of IP chemotherapy have confirmed that tumor volume is a very important determinant of the efficacy of IP chemotherapy. In patients with ovarian carcinoma, IP chemotherapy is more effective for patients whose largest tumor nodule is less than 2 cm and less effective when the nodules are larger [4]. Los et al. [5] reported studies done in a murine colon carcinoma showing that the advantage of an IP over an IV injection was limited to approximately 1.5 mm depth into the tumor from the surface and that a peritoneal-to-plasma AUC ratio of 12–15 produced a 1.7-fold increase in drug delivery to such nodules. Importantly, this study also demonstrated that even in nodules of just a few millimeters, the drug content of the tumor varied widely between nodules.

7.5
Intraperitoneal Drug Distribution

It is axiomatic that to enter a tumor nodule growing on the peritoneal surface, the intraperitoneally instilled drug must actually reach the nodule. Ovarian carcinomas characteristically produce adhesions that limit the free distribution of drug with the cavity. This was a major factor in the poor results obtained in early clinical trials that included patients with large volume disease [6, 7]. It often remains a problem even in patients in whom most or all of the visible disease has been surgically removed. The standard approach to trying to ensure that drug reaches all of the crevices within the peritoneal cavity is to instill drugs in large volumes (e.g., 1.4 L/m^2), since drugs instilled in small volumes do not distribute well even when the patient is repositioned from side to side.

7.6
Principles for the Selection of Drugs for Intraperitoneal Administration

Two key principles drive the selection of drugs for IP therapy. First, one would like to use drugs that have a very high peritoneal-to-plasma AUC ratio. Second, the drug should not produce damage to the peritoneal surface; the dose-limiting toxicity should be a result of the drug that enters the bloodstream rather than local toxicity of the drug in the cavity. Given the limitations of drug penetration, successful destruction of even small tumor nodules is likely to require repeated cycles of exposure to drug with each cycle removing the outermost layer of malignant cells. Thus drugs such as doxorubicin and mitoxantrone, which cause peritoneal inflammation with associated fibrosis and adhesion formation that limit drug distribution within the peritoneal cavity, are not useful for IP therapy. The use of a drug that does not produce chemical irritation of the peritoneal surface has the important advantage that the dose can be escalated to the point where the amount of drug leaking into the systemic circulation produces a plasma AUC equivalent to that which could be produced by an IV injection. This results in a situation where there is no compromise to the amount of drug being delivered to the tumor by capillary flow from the plasma compartment. In other words, if a drug has a high AUC ratio and does not produce local toxicity, for a given amount of systemic toxicity, one can obtain a substantially greater AUC for the surface of the tumor without reducing capillary drug delivery by using the IP rather than the IV route of injection. Actual measurements of the distribution of drugs in ovarian cancer nodules following IP vs. IV injections are very limited. However, it is reasonable to expect that the concurrent delivery of drug to a tumor nodule by both capillary flow from the vascular compartment and free surface diffusion from the peritoneal cavity will result in a more even distribution of drug within the nodule as well as an incremental increase in total drug exposure.

7.7
Pharmacokinetics of Intraperitoneally Administered Cisplatin, Carboplatin, and Paclitaxel

Cisplatin, carboplatin, and paclitaxel are currently the drugs most extensively used for IP therapy. Table 7.1 presents the pharmacokinetic parameters for these three agents summarized from representative studies among the many that have been reported [6, 8–10]. Cisplatin has an AUC ratio of 15 when drug levels were measured using an assay for those forms of the drug capable of reacting with a thio-containing molecule [6]. Studies of the pharmacokinetics of IP carboplatin are more limited, but its AUC ratio appears to be similar to that of cisplatin, as would be expected based on the similarity of their molecular characteristics. Paclitaxel behaves very differently. In spite of the fact that paclitaxel is much more lipid soluble and thus might be expected to diffuse across the peritoneal

Table 7.1 Pharmacokinetic parameters of cisplatin, carboplatin, and paclitaxel in the peritoneal cavity following injection by the intraperitoneal (IP) route

	Cisplatin	Carboplatin	Paclitaxel
$T_{1/2 \text{ peritoneum}}$ (h)	0.88		73.4
$Cl_{\text{peritoneum}}$ (L/m²/h)	1.4		0.0175
AUC ratio	15[a]	17[a]	996
Bioavailability (%)	100	100	46–53

[a]Filtrable Pt

membrane more readily, it has an AUC ratio in the range of 996 [10]. Why paclitaxel has such a long residence time in the peritoneal cavity is not entirely clear, but its high AUC ratio makes it of particular interest for use by the IP route.

It is important to note that a high peritoneal-to-plasma AUC ratio by itself is not sufficient to make a drug attractive, it must also be able to penetrate into the nodule from the free surface. Early studies of penetration of cisplatin and carboplatin in a rat colon cancer model were reported by Los et al. [5, 11]. Figure 7.2, reprinted from their work, shows that IP injection of cisplatin produced higher platinum content near the surface of the nodule than in the interior, whereas IV administration resulted in lower platinum levels at the edge but approximately equal levels in the deeper parts of the nodule. Marked heterogeneity of platinum levels was noted even within a small 3–5 mm nodule. While the more peripheral portions near the surface had generally higher levels than the center of the nodule, even near the edge there were sections where the platinum content was low. Figure 7.3 shows thatthe administration of carboplatin produces a different profile of drug penetration.

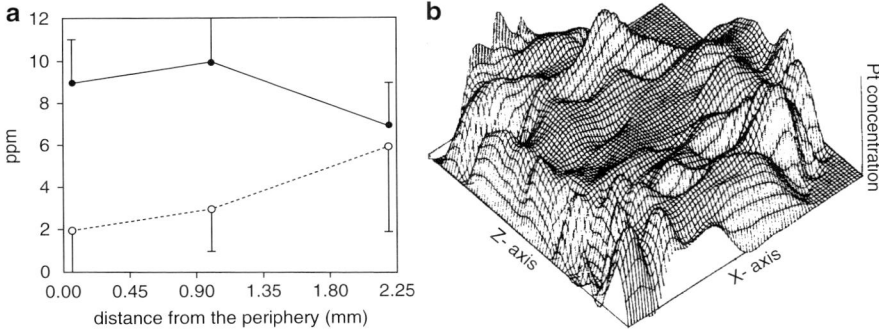

Fig. 7.2 (**a**) Platinum levels as a function of distance from the tumor nodule surface in rat treated with equal doses of cisplatin by the intraperitoneal (IP) (*closed circle*) and intravenous (IV) route (*open circle*). (**b**) Distribution of Pt in a representative 2–5 mm rat colon carcinoma nodule as determined by proton-induced X-ray emission (PIXE). Reproduced by permission from Los et al. [5]

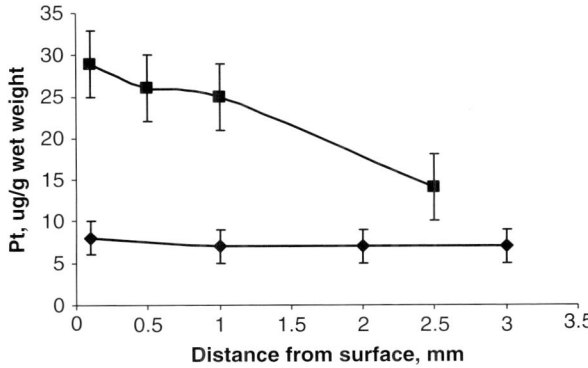

Fig. 7.3 Comparison of the penetration of cisplatin (*closed square*) and carboplatin (*closed diamond*) into rat colon carcinoma tumor nodules. Redrawn from Los et al. [11]

The platinum levels achieved are lower, but more importantly, the gradient from the surface to the center is much less steep for carboplatin than for cisplatin. The better penetration by carboplatin than by cisplatin has been confirmed in a more recent study that utilized a human ovarian cancer model grown in athymic mice [12]. Human 2008 cells expressing green fluorescent protein (GFP) were inoculated IP in nude athymic (nu/nu) mice. When small tumor nodules became visible by external imaging, a maximum tolerated dose of cisplatin, or either an equimolar or equitoxic dose of carboplatin, was injected IP. Cisplatin produced a 3.4-fold higher level of platinum in tumor nodules when compared to an equimolar dose of carboplatin ($p=0.02$). However, when cisplatin and carboplatin were injected at equitoxic doses, the tumor platinum levels were similar. Confirming the studies in the rat colon carcinoma model, the platinum content of equal-sized nodules was highly variable. Following injection of cisplatin, tumor platinum per mg decreased with increasing nodule size. In contrast, following injection of either equimolar or equitoxic doses, carboplatin tumor platinum per mg remained constant as nodule size increased ($p<0.0001$). These results suggest that IP carboplatin has comparable or better drug penetration when compared to cisplatin given at equitoxic doses and thus provide a rationale for replacing cisplatin with carboplatin in the IP treatment of patients with ovarian cancer. The better penetration of carboplatin is probably related to the fact that carboplatin is less reactive than cisplatin and is less susceptible to sequestration by binding to extracellular matrix molecules or by uptake into the outer cell layers of the tumor nodule than cisplatin.

7.8
Neutralizing Agents

The availability of competitive neutralizing agents for methotrexate and cisplatin prompted early studies of their use to enhance the therapeutic index of IP therapy. The concept is that if one could neutralize the drug reaching the systemic compartment by injecting the neutralizing agent IV concurrently with the IP administration of the chemotherapeutic agent, one could give even larger doses IP and thus attain higher concentration gradients favoring drug penetration and an overall increase in AUC. Since the neutralizing or rescue agent can get into the tumor via capillary flow and can potentially enter the peritoneal cavity, this strategy depends critically on the concentration of the chemotherapeutic and protective agents actually attained in the tumor, as well as the protective agent being a competitive rather than noncompetitive antagonist. Ideally, the neutralizing or rescue agent should be one whose ability to block the toxicity of the chemotherapeutic agent is overcome by relatively small increases in the latter's concentration. Early studies explored the use of systemically administered leucovorin in combination with intraperitoneally administered methotrexate [13]. These studies were based on the observation that these two drugs are competitive with each other, such that a concentration of leucovorin sufficient to block the effects of the low concentration of methotrexate found in the blood would not be expected to be adequate to offset the effect of the much higher concentrations of methotrexate in the peritoneal cavity and entering the tumor nodule by free surface penetration [13].

Another approach that has been explored involves the use of a neutralizing agent that reduces the toxicity of the active agent to the most sensitive normal tissue in the body. Thiosulfate is a competitive antagonist of cisplatin; it reacts with cisplatin to produce a complex that remains soluble, but is no longer toxic to either the kidneys or the tumor. When cisplatin is injected IP and thiosulfate IV, the concentration of thiosulfate in the plasma is still too low to produce much neutralization of cisplatin because the rate of reaction between the two is slower than the clearance of cisplatin by reaction with plasma proteins. However, thiosulfate is extensively concentrated in the kidneys where its concentration is then high enough to provide excellent protection [6]. This approach limits concern that the neutralizing agent reaching the tumor nodule by capillary flow would limit the activity of the chemotherapeutic agent.

7.9
Strategies for Improving Drug Penetration

One approach to increasing drug penetration is to increase the pressure gradient between the free surface of the tumor nodule and the interior. Several groups have explored simply increasing the intra-abdominal pressure. Using a rat colon carcinoma model, Esquis et al. [14] found that increasing the intra-abdominal pressure to 22 mg Hg during a 1 h exposure to IP cisplatin increased platinum levels in 0.5–3 mm serosal nodules by approximately 1.6-fold. This strategy is likely to be problematic in patients due to the fact that increasing abdominal pressure impairs venous return to the right heart.

A second approach is to reduce tumor blood flow by administering IP epinephrine. In a preclinical study using a colon carcinomatosis model, IP epinephrine was found to enhance platinum levels in 2–5 mm tumor nodules by up to 3.7-fold [15]. A phase I trial of this approach utilized 100 mg of cisplatin administered IP over 2 h in fluid containing progressively higher concentrations of epinephrine [16]. Even at a concentration of 5 mg/L, epinephrine produced few adverse events, and an epinephrine peritoneal-to-plasma concentration ratio of greater than 3,000 was attained by the end of the instillation. A third approach is to decrease tumor blood flow using a drug that interferes with the function of vascular endothelial growth factor (VEGF) or its receptor. A recent study of the effect of bevacizumab on the penetration of intraperitoneally administered topotecan demonstrated a 6.3-fold increase in tumor drug level in an ovarian carcinoma xenograft model [17]. In this study bevacizumab was given twice weekly starting three and a half weeks before a 72 h IP infusion of topotecan. There was no effect of bevacizumab on the plasma pharmacokinetics of topotecan, and bevacizumab did not increase tumor topotecan levels when it was given subcutaneously instead of intraperitoneally. The bevacizumab-induced increase in tumor topotecan level was accompanied by an approximate doubling of survival in this model. A similar increase in survival was attained when bevacizumab was given with cisplatin, although the impact of the antibody on tumor cisplatin levels was not assessed. The fact that bevacizumab by itself has promising activity in initial clinical trials in ovarian cancer [18] makes this approach to increasing drug penetration of immediate clinical interest and raises the question of whether similar results can be attained with tyrosine kinase inhibitors that block VEGF receptor signaling.

In principle, drug penetration should be increased simply by keeping the concentration of the chemotherapeutic agent in the peritoneal cavity at a very high level for a long period of time. This is only achievable with drugs that have very high steady-state peritoneal-to-plasma concentration ratios, such as those with rapid hepatic detoxification or very rapid plasma clearance. In such cases, it is possible to maintain cytotoxic concentrations in the peritoneal cavity under circumstances where the plasma concentrations are so low that there is little systemic toxicity. This approach was examined in phase I and II trials of cytarabine and fluorodeoxyuridine that produced some promising results, which have not yet been adequately followed up [19–21]. Gemcitabine has now also been shown to have a very high peritoneal-to-plasma AUC ratio (791–847) [22, 23] and it is a candidate for use in this strategy.

Another approach to increasing drug penetration is to deposit particles capable of slowly releasing drugs in the peritoneal cavity. The hypothesis is that cell-sized particles might be distributed to the same locations in the cavity as the tumor cells. A first-generation paclitaxel-loaded particle failed in a phase I trial due to a foreign body reaction to the particle [24]. However, several other paclitaxel-loaded particles [25, 26] and a cisplatin-loaded particle [27] have produced favorable results in preclinical tumor models. Several attempts have been made to target particles to the surface of tumor nodules using peptides that bind to receptors expressed at higher levels on the ovarian cancer cells than the mesothelium. The avidity of such peptides is markedly increased when they are multimerized on the surface of the particle [28]. An arginine–glycine–aspartic acid (RGD) peptide capable of binding to tumor integrins, attached to a chelating group carrying a radionuclide, has demonstrated antitumor activity in an animal model of ovarian cancer [29].

Finally, one of the challenges with the use of IP cisplatin is that this drug triggers the downregulation of its own influx transporter [30]. Studies from several different laboratories have now established that the major copper influx transporter, CTR1, controls the influx of cisplatin, carboplatin, and oxaliplatin [31, 32]. However, exposure of tumor cells to cisplatin causes ubiquitination and proteosomal degradation of CTR1, which rapidly limits continued uptake of the drug [30]. Recent preclinical studies have shown that blocking proteosomal degradation prevents the cisplatin-induced destruction of CTR1 [33], and that this results in cytotoxic synergy as well as enhanced cisplatin uptake and penetration in vitro and in vivo [34]. The clinically available proteosome inhibitor, bortezomib, was also shown to have a highly favorable peritoneal-to-plasma AUC ratio in a murine model of ovarian cancer [34], and the combination of IP cisplatin and bortezomib is an attractive approach to enhancing drug penetration in patients. A phase I trial of intraperitoneally administered bortezomid followed by carboplatin is currently under development.

References

1. Trimble EL, Christian MC (2006) Intraperitoneal chemotherapy for women with advanced epithelial ovarian carcinoma. Gynecol Oncol 100:3–4
2. Dedrick RL, Myers CE, Bungay PM, DeVita VT Jr (1978) Pharmacokinetic rationale for peritoneal drug administration in the treatment of ovarian cancer. Cancer Treat Rep 62:1–11

3. Dedrick RL, Flessner MF (1997) Pharmacokinetic problems in peritoneal drug administration: tissue penetration and surface exposure. J Natl Cancer Inst 89:480–487
4. Howell SB, Zimm S, Markman M, Abramson IS, Cleary S, Lucas WE, Weiss RJ (1987) Long-term survival of advanced refractory ovarian carcinoma patients with small-volume disease treated with intraperitoneal chemotherapy. J Clin Oncol 5:1607–1612
5. Los G, Mutsaers PH, Lenglet WJ, Baldew GS, McVie JG (1990) Platinum distribution in intraperitoneal tumors after intraperitoneal cisplatin treatment. Cancer Chemother Pharmacol 25:389–394
6. Howell SB, Pfeifle CL, Wung WE, Olshen RA, Lucas WE, Yon JL, Green M (1982) Intraperitoneal cisplatin with systemic thiosulfate protection. Ann Intern Med 97:845–851
7. Kirmani S, Braly PS, McClay EF, Saltzstein SL, Plaxe SC, Kim S, Cates C, Howell SB (1994) A comparison of intravenous versus intraperitoneal chemotherapy for the initial treatment of ovarian cancer. Gynecol Oncol 54:338–344
8. Elferink F, Vander Vijgh WJF, Klein I, Ten Bokkel Huinink WW, Dubbleman R, McVie JG (1988) Pharmacokinetics of carboplatin after intraperitoneal administration. Cancer Chemother Pharmacol 21:4157–4160
9. Howell SB, Pfeifle CE, Wung WE, Olshen RA (1983) Intraperitoneal cis-diamminedichloroplatinum with systemic thiosulfate protection. Cancer Res 43:1426–1431
10. Markman M, Rowinsky E, Hakes T, Reichman B, Jones W, Lewis JL Jr, Rubin S, Curtin J, Barakat R, Phillips M, Hurowitz L, Almadrones L, Hoskins W (1992) Phase I trial of intraperitoneal taxol: a gynecologic oncology group study. J Clin Oncol 10:1485–1491
11. Los G, Verdegaal EM, Mutsaers PH, McVie JG (1991) Penetration of carboplatin and cisplatin into rat peritoneal tumor nodules after intraperitoneal chemotherapy. Cancer Chemother Pharmacol 28:159–165
12. Jandial DD, Farshchi-Heydari S, Pu M, Messer K, Howell SB (2009) Tumor platinum concentration following intraperitoneal administration of cisplatin versus carboplatin in an ovarian cancer model. Gynecol Oncol 115:362–6. PMID: 19775736; PMCID: PMC2707998
13. Howell SB, Chu BB, Wung WE, Metha BM, Mendelsohn J (1981) Long-duration intracavitary infusion of methotrexate with systemic leucovorin protection in patients with malignant effusions. J Clin Invest 67:1161–1170
14. Esquis P, Consolo D, Magnin G, Pointaire P, Moretto P, Ynsa MD, Beltramo JL, Drogoul C, Simonet M, Benoit L, Rat P, Chauffert B (2006) High intra-abdominal pressure enhances the penetration and antitumor effect of intraperitoneal cisplatin on experimental peritoneal carcinomatosis. Ann Surg 244:106–112
15. Favoulet P, Magnin G, Guilland JC, Beltramo JL, Osmak L, Benoit L, Rat P, Douvier S, Duvillard C, Chauffert B (2001) Pre-clinical study of the epinephrine-cisplatin association for the treatment of intraperitoneal carcinomatosis. Eur J Surg Oncol 27:59–64
16. Molucon-Chabrot C, Isambert N, Benoit L, Zanetta S, Fraisse J, Guilland JC, Royer B, Monin-Baroille P, Flesch M, Fargeot P, Coudert B, Mayer F, Fumoleau P, Chauffert B (2006) Feasibility of using intraperitoneal epinephrine and cisplatin in patients with advanced peritoneal carcinomatosis. Anticancer Drugs 17:1211–1217
17. Shah DK, Shin BS, Veith J, Toth K, Bernacki RJ, Balthasar JP (2009) Use of an anti-vascular endothelial growth factor antibody in a pharmacokinetic strategy to increase the efficacy of intraperitoneal chemotherapy. J Pharmacol Exp Ther 329:580–591
18. Burger RA (2007) Experience with bevacizumab in the management of epithelial ovarian cancer. J Clin Oncol 25:2902–2908
19. King ME, Pfeifle CE, Howell SB (1984) Intraperitoneal cytosine arabinoside therapy in ovarian carcinoma. J Clin Oncol 2:662–669
20. Kirmani S, Zimm S, Cleary SM, Mowry J, Howell SB (1990) Extremely prolonged continuous intraperitoneal infusion of cytosine arabinoside. Cancer Chemother Pharmacol 25:454–458

21. Muggia FM, Jeffers S, Muderspach L, Roman L, Rosales R, Groshen S, Safra T, Morrow CP (1997) Phase I/II study of intraperitoneal floxuridine and platinums (cisplatin and/or carboplatin). Gynecol Oncol 66:290–294

22. Morgan RJ Jr, Synold TW, Xi B, Lim D, Shibata S, Margolin K, Schwarz RE, Leong L, Somlo G, Twardowski P, Yen Y, Chow W, Tetef M, Lin P, Paz B, Koczywas M, Wagman L, Chu D, Frankel P, Stalter S, Doroshow JH (2007) Phase I trial of intraperitoneal gemcitabine in the treatment of advanced malignancies primarily confined to the peritoneal cavity. Clin Cancer Res 13:1232–1237

23. Sabbatini P, Aghajanian C, Leitao M, Venkatraman E, Anderson S, Dupont J, Dizon D, O'Flaherty C, Bloss J, Chi D, Spriggs D (2004) Intraperitoneal cisplatin with intraperitoneal gemcitabine in patients with epithelial ovarian cancer: results of a phase I/II trial. Clin Cancer Res 10:2962–2967

24. Armstrong DK, Fleming GF, Markman M, Bailey HH (2006) A phase I trial of intraperitoneal sustained-release paclitaxel microspheres (Paclimer) in recurrent ovarian cancer: a Gynecologic Oncology Group study. Gynecol Oncol 103:391–396

25. Tsai M, Lu Z, Wang J, Yeh TK, Wientjes MG, Au JL (2007) Effects of carrier on disposition and antitumor activity of intraperitoneal paclitaxel. Pharm Res 24:1691–1701

26. Vassileva V, Grant J, De Souza R, Allen C, Piquette-Miller M (2007) Novel biocompatible intraperitoneal drug delivery system increases tolerability and therapeutic efficacy of paclitaxel in a human ovarian cancer xenograft model. Cancer Chemother Pharmacol 60:907–914

27. Xu P, Van Kirk EA, Murdoch WJ, Zhan Y, Isaak DD, Radosz M, Shen Y (2006) Anticancer efficacies of cisplatin-releasing pH-responsive nanoparticles. Biomacromolecules 7:829–835

28. Carlson CB, Mowery P, Owen RM, Dykhuizen EC, Kiessling LL (2007) Selective tumor cell targeting using low-affinity, multivalent interactions. ACS Chem Biol 2:119–127

29. Dijkgraaf I, Kruijtzer JA, Frielink C, Corstens FH, Oyen WJ, Liskamp RM, Boerman OC (2007) Alpha v beta 3 integrin-targeting of intraperitoneally growing tumors with a radiolabeled RGD peptide. Int J Cancer 120:605–610

30. Holzer AK, Katano K, Klomp LW, Howell SB (2004) Cisplatin rapidly down-regulates its own influx transporter hCTR1 in cultured human ovarian carcinoma cells. Clin Cancer Res 10:6744–6749

31. Holzer AK, Samimi G, Katano K, Naerdemann W, Lin X, Safaei R, Howell SB (2004) The copper influx transporter human copper transport protein 1 regulates the uptake of cisplatin in human ovarian carcinoma cells. Mol Pharmacol 66:817–823

32. Larson CA. Blair BG, Safaei R, Howell SB (2009) The role of the mammalian copper transporter 1 in the cellular accumulation of platinum-based drugs. Mol Pharmacol 75:324–330

33. Holzer AK, Howell SB (2006) The internalization and degradation of human copper transporter 1 following cisplatin exposure. Cancer Res 66:10944–10952

34. Jandial DD. Farshchi-Heydari S, Larson CA, Elliot GI, Wrasidlo WJ, Howell SB (2009) Enhanced delivery of cisplatin to intraperitoneal ovarian carcinomas mediated by the effects of bortezomib on the human copper transporter 1. Clin Cancer Res 15:553–560

Administration Guidelines for Intraperitoneal Chemotherapy for Ovarian Cancer

8

Deborah K. Armstrong

8.1
Introduction

Successful delivery of intraperitoneal (IP) chemotherapy requires a multidisciplinary team with both expertise and dedication to optimizing the outcome from IP delivery. In general, this will require a sufficient volume of candidates for IP therapy to preserve expertise, and maintain skills and experience among clinic staff. Staffing for IP treatment requires a gynecologic oncologist with experience in optimal cytoreductive surgery and placement of IP ports, either a gynecologic oncologist or medical oncologist with experience in prescribing IP chemotherapy and managing IP toxicities, and oncology nurses with experience in administering IP chemotherapy and recognizing IP port problems. In addition, it is helpful to have diagnostic and interventional imaging staff familiar with IP catheters to assist in evaluating port problems.

Patients receiving IP chemotherapy require more time and resources than a similar patient receiving only intravenous (IV) chemotherapy. In the outpatient setting, a woman receiving IP chemotherapy needs to be able to recline on a bed or stretcher. In addition, IP infusions usually last longer than comparable IV infusions. These requirements may affect both staffing and equipment needs. If a 24-h infusion of paclitaxel is conducted in the hospital, rather than in the outpatient setting, additional in-patient beds need to be available for that purpose. It should be noted that centers with expertise in giving IP chemotherapy identify consistency in orders, port placement, chemotherapy delivery, and management of toxicities as the most important factors in the success of IP chemotherapy programs [1].

8.2
Selection of Patients for IP Chemotherapy

The three published randomized North American trials demonstrating a survival benefit for the use of IP therapy have all used cisplatin IP as initial therapy in patients with

D.K. Armstrong
Johns Hopkins Kimmel Cancer Center, 1650 Orleans Street, Baltimore, MD 21231, USA
e-mail: darmstro@jhmi.edu

D.S. Alberts et al. (eds.), *Intraperitoneal Therapy for Ovarian Cancer*,
DOI: 10.1007/978-3-642-12130-2_8, © Springer-Verlag Berlin Heidelberg 2010

optimally debulked stage III disease [2–4]. While the definition of optimal residual disease differed in the trials, peritoneal drugs are not expected to be able to fully penetrate large tumors [5]. Thus, IP therapy is most appropriate for patients with low volume residual disease after initial surgery. In addition, patients need to be good candidates for cisplatin. Those with significant preexisting neuropathy or renal dysfunction may not be well-suited to receive cisplatin either IP or IV. In addition, patients with cardiovascular problems such as congestive heart failure may not tolerate the predicted fluid shifts related to both pre- and postcisplatin hydration and the absorption of IP fluids, and thus may not be well served by the use of IP cisplatin. Patients with significant peritoneal adhesions may not tolerate IP treatments due to pain and poor delivery of IP fluids and drugs to all peritoneal surfaces. Thus the finding of significant adhesions at initial cytoreductive surgery is a relative contraindication to IP therapy. Finally, patients with postoperative infections or who experience complications of abdominal healing may not tolerate IP therapy, at least until these problems resolve [6].

8.3
Positioning the Patient

Women should be placed supine on a stretcher, gurney, or bed. The head of the bed should be no higher than 30° to prevent dislocation of the right-angled needle during infusion. A flat or Trendelenburg position during IP infusion may result in increased pressure on the diaphragm causing respiratory compromise. Once the IP port has been accessed, patients should not ambulate. Therefore, the patient should be in an area that ensures privacy for use of the bedpan, if necessary.

8.4
Premedications Before IP Therapy

In addition to IP port access, all patients receiving IP therapy should have peripheral IV access for premedications, hydration, antiemetics, and for the rapid treatment of hypersensitivity reactions. It is critical that patients who will be receiving IP cisplatin have IV hydration before and after cisplatin, in a manner similar to patients receiving IV cisplatin. Many have incorrectly assumed that the IP instillate can substitute for the IV hydration. However, because the absorption of IP fluid is variable and unpredictable, IV hydration should always be used to ensure adequate renal perfusion before, during, and after the administration of IP cisplatin. High-dose cisplatin, as is used in IP treatment, requires aggressive antiemetic therapy [7]. This should include an NK1 antagonist such as aprepitant or fosaprepitant, a 5-HT3 receptor antagonist such as palonosetron, dolasetron, or ondansetron, and dexamethasone [7]. Treatment with lorazepam can decrease anxiety as well as help control nausea. Use of an H2 receptor antagonist or a proton pump inhibitor can also benefit patients who experience gastrointestinal (GI) reflux symptoms or other GI distress with treatment. Patients who are receiving IP paclitaxel should have the same systemic premedications that are used for IV paclitaxel.

8.5
Accessing the IP Port

Placement of the IP port has been previously covered in the Chap. 6 by Walker. IP therapy for ovarian cancer is usually accomplished using a semipermanent catheter rather than repeated placement of temporary catheters [8]. Two types of semipermanent catheters can be used; external catheters or implanted catheters. The least commonly used are the external catheters such as Tenckhoff. Most physicians prefer subcutaneously implanted catheters such as the Mediport. The latter require no day-to-day care by the patient and allow for ease of showering and even swimming. If an external catheter is used, only the appropriate, approved connectors should be utilized for accessing the catheter to minimize the risk of leaking or of damaging the connector.

For subcutaneous ports, pretreatment with a topical anesthetic cream, such as EMLA 2.5% 1 h before port access will minimize discomfort for the patient. IP devices should always be accessed using an aseptic technique. Since the sterility of the topical anesthetic cream cannot be guaranteed, it is important that the access site be cleaned and prepped *after* the use of anesthetic cream. A right angle needle, such as the Huber needle, provides the greatest stability once the port is accessed, and is preferred. The needle should be secured in place with a sterile dressing and tape. It is important to use a needle that is of sufficient gauge (usually 19–20 gauge) to allow timely flow, and adequate length (typically 1.5–2.0 in.) to safely access the port. A longer needle helps prevent infiltration and increases the ease of administration of IP fluids. A small volume normal saline flush is usually used at the time of catheter placement. It is not common to be able to withdraw peritoneal fluid, even after administration of 1–2 L, from IP access needles. Thus, unlike IV ports, the inability to withdraw fluid from an accessed IP port is common and is not a contraindication to treatment.

8.6
Delivery of IP Therapy

It should be guaranteed that the needle is properly placed and the flow of fluids into the IP cavity is adequate before any chemotherapy is administered through the port. For this reason, it is advisable to start with at least 500–1,000 cc of isotonic fluid (usually normal saline) to be infused first, without the ordered chemotherapy agent. This approach allows for the identification of potential problems such as infiltration, extravasation, significant resistance to flow, patient intolerance, or catheter malfunction using a solution without the chemotherapy agent. Fluids that will be infused IP should be warmed to body temperature before infusion. Cold or even room temperature fluids can cause cramping, abdominal pain, and burning. Warming should be done using a method that will not result in overheated fluids. K-packs or blood or blanket warmers are commonly used methods for warming. Since the potency and safety of most chemotherapeutic agents at temperatures above room temperature have not been well studied, it is advised to warm fluid for IP administration without the chemotherapy drug added.

A total of 1,500–2,000 cc of fluid is usually given IP, which allows for adequate distribution within the peritoneal cavity. The chemotherapy for IP administration can be either diluted in the last 500–1,000 cc of IP fluid, or administered as a concentrate after 1,500–2,000 cc of fluid has been given IP. Pressurized IV pumps should not be used for IP administration of fluids or chemotherapy. Rather, all IP administration should be delivered via gravity.

As long as there is sufficient fluid already in the peritoneal cavity, there is no benefit in the slow delivery of IP chemotherapy; thus, most clinicians find it the easiest to give a bolus of chemotherapy at the completion of IP fluid.

After IP administration, the concentration of drugs within the peritoneal cavity will change depending on the rapidity of absorption of IP fluid, and the size and solubility of the IP administered drug. For most drugs used for the treatment of ovarian cancer, IP and systemic kinetics have been carefully evaluated. It bears repeating that outside of the study setting, no drugs should be used IP unless they have been well studied and the kinetics, tolerability, and efficacy have been clearly documented. Some agents used IV can cause severe peritoneal irritation (e.g., doxorubicin). Others may be absorbed so quickly as to make IP administration unnecessary. Most chemotherapeutic agents undergo little metabolism in the peritoneal cavity [5].

Once IP administration is completed, the access needle should be removed and a pressure dressing applied. This will help prevent back leakage from the port into subcutaneous tissues. The patient should be instructed to remove the pressure dressing after 24 h. After IP infusion is complete, patients may begin a "turning protocol." This protocol may direct turning at 10–15 min intervals for up to 2 h. However, if IP fluid volumes of 1,500–2,000 cc are used, adequate distribution within the peritoneal cavity is assured and it is not likely that turning provides any additional value.

After all planned IP treatments are completed, the IP catheter does not serve any useful purpose and should be removed. The noncuffed silicone ports can usually be easily removed as a minor surgical procedure.

8.7
Trouble-Shooting Problems with IP Administration

If the port cannot be accessed, an imaging study should be done to evaluate whether the port has "flipped" resulting in the port access site not facing the skin. If the port has been placed over the lower anterior ribs, a lateral chest X-ray will sometimes be sufficient to make this diagnosis. Optimally, a flipped port access device should be repositioned and resutured or replaced surgically. If the port has been placed over the lower ribs, it should not be too deep to be accessed. However, ports placed in the lower quadrants, without a firm surface behind them can sometimes be too deep in the subcutaneous tissues to easily palpate and access. In that case, fluoroscopy is the best means to evaluate the port and direct the needle.

Infusion times will vary from patient to patient. Slow flow can often be remedied by reaccessing and flushing the port. If the patient experiences sharp pain, the infusion should be stopped and the attending physician should be notified. A dye study may be ordered to assess the patency of the port and catheter. It is critical that a dye that will not cause peritoneal irritation is used. Access to fluoroscopy during the dye study is optimal as this can quickly diagnose extravasation (e.g., if the catheter has become dislodged from the access port or has cracked) or establish whether the dye is reaching the peritoneal cavity. This methodology can also help determine if adhesions or loculations are present, such as if dye is flowing back along the port tract or if the catheter has perforated the GI tract. If port malfunction cannot be rectified in a short period of time, alternative IV chemotherapy should be given according to the treating physician's directions.

Mild complaints of pain with IP infusion can usually be managed with analgesics or narcotics. Orders for both IV and oral pain medications should accompany standard IP treatment orders so that patient discomfort can be addressed quickly.

8.8
Long-Term Tolerability of IP Chemotherapy

The main barriers to continuing IP therapy throughout the planned treatment arise from one of the following three problems: those related to the IP catheter and access device; those related to abdominal pain with infusion; and those related to cisplatin toxicities. Close attention to these issues with early intervention is critical, but if problems are adequately addressed, it is clear that more patients will be able to complete the planned IP therapy.

For patients who have difficulty with abdominal pain, verifying the temperature of the infusate, decreasing the rate of infusion, or using a smaller volume may be sufficient to address the problem. Some patients benefit from additional IV fluids and antiemetics 3–5 days after cisplatin. Building in a clinic visit and nurse assessment with the first cycle is reassuring to patients and can frequently avoid later or cumulative problems. Close attention to renal function and electrolytes and dose reduction of cisplatin for subjective as well as objective signs of poor tolerance is also prudent.

The IP catheter is a foreign body that can become infected. In addition, the increased intensity of some IP regimens increases the risk of myelosuppression and its complications. If such intense regimens are used, prophylactic white blood cell growth factors can be used. While these growth factors should not be used concurrent with IV chemotherapy, they can be used throughout the time when IP paclitaxel is given, without evidence of cumulative myelosuppression [9]. This is likely due to the very small amount of IP paclitaxel that is absorbed into the systemic circulation.

8.9
Summary

In summary, IP administration of chemotherapy for the treatment of ovarian cancer is a process that, like any other medical process, benefits from experience and dedication of the treating medical staff. Careful attention to the details of safe administration and good communication are critical to understand both the objective and subjective patient experience. Adherence to these guidelines will lead to an improved outcome for both patient and staff.

References

1. Trimble EL, Thompson S, Christian MC, Minasian L (2008) Intraperitoneal chemotherapy for women with epithelial ovarian cancer. Oncologist 13(4):403–409
2. Alberts DS, Liu PY, Hannigan EV, O'Toole R, Williams SD, Young JA, Franklin EW, Clarke-Pearson DL, Malviya VK, DuBeshter B (1996) Intraperitoneal cisplatin plus intravenous cyclophosphamide versus intravenous cisplatin plus intravenous cyclophosphamide for stage III ovarian cancer. N Engl J Med 335(26):1950–1955
3. Armstrong DK, Bundy B, Wenzel L, Huang HQ, Baergen R, Lele S, Copeland LJ, Walker JL, Burger RA (2006) Gynecologic Oncology Group. Intraperitoneal cisplatin and paclitaxel in ovarian cancer. N Engl J Med 354(1):34–43
4. Markman M, Bundy BN, Alberts DS, Fowler JM, Clark-Pearson DL, Carson LF, Wadler S, Sickel J (2001) Phase III trial of standard-dose intravenous cisplatin plus paclitaxel versus moderately high-dose carboplatin followed by intravenous paclitaxel and intraperitoneal cisplatin in small-volume stage III ovarian carcinoma: an intergroup study of the Gynecologic Oncology Group, Southwestern Oncology Group, and Eastern Cooperative Oncology Group. J Clin Oncol 19(4):1001–1007
5. Howell SB (2008) Pharmacologic principles of intraperitoneal chemotherapy for the treatment of ovarian cancer. Int J Gynecol Cancer 18(Suppl 1):20–25
6. Walker JL, Armstrong DK, Huang HQ, Fowler J, Webster K, Burger RA, Clarke-Pearson D (2006) Intraperitoneal catheter outcomes in a phase III trial of intravenous versus intraperitoneal chemotherapy in optimal stage III ovarian and primary peritoneal cancer: a Gynecologic Oncology Group Study. Gynecol Oncol 100(1):27–32
7. Morgan RJ Jr, Alvarez RD, Armstrong DK, Boston B, Chen LM, Copeland L, Fowler J, Gaffney DK, Gershenson D, Greer BE, Grigsby PW, Havrilesky LJ, Johnston C, Lancaster JM, Lele S, Matulonis U, O'Malley D, Ozols RF, Remmenga SW, Sabbatini P, Schink J, Neng N (2008) National comprehensive cancer network. Ovarian cancer. Clinical practice guidelines in oncology. J Natl Compl Canc Netw 6(8):766–94. PMID: 18926089
8. Markman M, Walker JL (2006) Intraperitoneal chemotherapy of ovarian cancer: a review, with a focus on practical aspects of treatment. J Clin Oncol 24(6):988–994, Epub 2006
9. Alberts DS, Delforge A (2006) Maximizing the delivery of intraperitoneal therapy while minimizing drug toxicity and maintaining quality of life. Semin Oncol 33(6 Suppl 12):S8–S17

Novel Drugs for Intraperitoneal Therapy for Ovarian Cancer

9

Boris Kobrinsky and Franco Muggia

9.1
Introduction

When the concept of a pharmacologically based administration of anticancer drugs by the IP route was first introduced by Dedrick et al. [1] at the National Institutes of Health, a sequence of clinical studies were initiated at the Medicine and Pharmacology Branches of the Division of Cancer Treatment, National Cancer Institute (NCI). The drugs that were initially studied were methotrexate [2], doxorubicin [3, 4], and 5-fluorouracil [5–7]. Subsequently, a number of other groups joined in evaluating the IP administration of drugs including University of California, San Diego (UCSD), the Netherlands Cancer Institute (NKI), New York University (NYU), Memorial Sloan-Kettering Cancer Center (MSKCC), Roswell Park Memorial Institute (RPMI), and the University of Southern California (USC). Table 9.1 summarizes the salient findings of a number of these and other drugs such as the platinums [8–11], alkylating drugs [12–14], antimetabolites [15–19], taxanes [20, 21], and topoisomerase-interacting drugs [22–24] that subsequently underwent phase I and pharmacologic studies.

These initial phase I studies led to a number of combination studies to take advantage of possible additivity or synergy with platinum drugs. Because the platinum drugs had shown particular activity in the treatment of ovarian cancer, they were seen as likely candidates for IP drug administration [12, 22, 25–27]. Publication of promising therapeutic results encouraged the widespread use of IP treatment for "small volume" ovarian cancer present in the peritoneal cavity. To explore the use of IP therapy in the second-line setting of patients with small volume disease, 31 patients were enrolled to a phase II study following the completion of front-line cisplatin-based therapy [26]. Disease status was determined at "second-look" surgery coupled with surgical cytoreduction. Patients were then treated with second-line IP treatment, followed by a "third-look" open laparotomy that determined the response to treatment. Some response was seen among patients with small

B. Kobrinsky and F. Muggia (✉)
NYU Cancer Institute, NYU Langone Medical Center,
New York, NY 10016, USA
e-mail: franco.muggia@nyumc.org

D.S. Alberts et al. (eds.), *Intraperitoneal Therapy for Ovarian Cancer*,
DOI: 10.1007/978-3-642-12130-2_9, © Springer-Verlag Berlin Heidelberg 2010

Table 9.1 Cytotoxic drugs that have undergone phase I/II evaluation by the intraperitoneal (IP) route

Agent [reference]	Median AUC[a] ratio IP/plasma	Local toxicity	Systemic dose-limiting toxicities/other
Cisplatin [9, 10]	12	+/−	Emesis, renal
Carboplatin [11]	10	-	Bone marrow
Melphalan [13]	65	-	Bone marrow
Thiotepa [12]	4	-	Bone marrow
Mitomycin [14]	32	+++	Peritonitis, bone marrow
Doxorubicin [3, 4]	400	++	Peritonitis
Mitoxantrone [87]	1,400	++	Peritonitis, catheter occlusions
Methotrexate [2]	92	+	Bone marrow
Fluorouracil [5–7]	376	++	Peritonitis, bone marrow
Floxuridine [15, 18, 19]	>1,000	-	Stomatitis, bone marrow
Cytarabine [16]	300–1,000	++	Bone marrow
Etoposide [23, 24]	65	-	Alopecia, bone marrow
Paclitaxel [20]	1,000	++	Abdominal pain, neuropathy
Docetaxel [21]	152	+/-	Bone marrow
Gemcitabine [17]	847	-	Bone marrow
Topotecan [22]	100	-	Bone marrow
Irinotecan [53]	Not published	-	Not published
Oxaliplatin [8]	25	+++	Thrombocytopenia, abdominal pain[b]

[a]Area under the curve (concentration × time)
[b]Personal communication, Memorial Sloan Kettering phase I trial (L Saltz)
[c]Trial at USC (S Iqbal and A Elkhoueiry)

volume disease. In order to confirm or refute these reports, in the late 1980s, the Gynecologic Oncology Group (GOG) began a series of similarly structured Phase II studies of IP administered drugs (GOG 0102 series; Table 9.2) [12, 28–32]. A general conclusion from these studies was that phase III randomized trials were required, and that the best setting for IP therapy would be in first-line treatment. This conclusion led to cooperative group trials GOG 0104, GOG 0114, and GOG 0172, which are described elsewhere in this volume. Specific findings from these phase III studies encouraged the development of IP cisplatin and IP paclitaxel in the front-line setting. Previous results had been regarded as disappointing because of the initially high expectations with the use of IP drugs in the recurrent

Table 9.2 Gynecologic Oncology Group (GOG) IP phase II studies [33]

IP regimen	Protocol number
Cisplatin + 5-fluorouracil [30]	GOG 0102B
Cisplatin + alpha-interferon (α-IFN) [31]	GOG 0102C
Cisplatin + etoposide [32]	GOG 0102E
α-IFN [29]	GOG 0102F
Cisplatin + thioTepa [12]	GOG 0102G
α-IFN alternating with cisplatin [28]	GOG 0102N

setting, the difficulty in interpreting endpoints such as objective response at "third look," and the relatively short progression-free survival of second-line IP therapy.

In this chapter, we review the status of drugs and drug regimens that may be ready for further clinical study, as well as point to some exciting new directions in the search for more active IP regimens.

9.2
Therapeutic IP Approaches: The Next Generation Carboplatin

The use of IP carboplatin in lieu of cisplatin has been the subject of ample debate [33]. Initial clinical studies of IP carboplatin established its pharmacologic advantage and were associated with therapeutic responses [11]. Subsequently, studies in Japan established the safety and therapeutic effects of IP carboplatin in the first-line setting combined with IV paclitaxel [34]. The GOG has also piloted the use of carboplatin in combination with IP and IV paclitaxel, and has demonstrated the feasibility of such an approach. This approach is tested in combination with bevacizumab as an arm of GOG 0252, a phase III study comparing three IP therapy regimens, which began enrollment in the summer of 2009.

9.2.1
Oxaliplatin

Preclinical studies have been done with oxaliplatin in adult pigs, and its pharmacology was established using both closed (laparoscopically inserted perfusion drains) and open laparotomy system used in chemo-hyperthermia (HIPEC). These studies have shown that the closed system significantly enhances the clearance of the drug out of the peritoneal cavity, resulting in higher blood levels [35]. Interest has increased since clinical studies using oxaliplatin-based HIPEC in colorectal cancer performed in France nearly 10 years ago yielded striking results [36]. On the other hand, attempts to deliver this IP oxaliplatin in patients without anesthesia were terminated early because of the severe abdominal pain experienced by all patients upon drug administration (Saltz L, personal communication).

Fagotti et al. [37] performed a single institution pilot study of oxaliplatin-based HIPEC in 25 platinum-sensitive patients who had either a recurrence at least 6 months after the last platinum-based therapy or a second recurrence, but remained platinum sensitive. Seventy-six percent of this study population had diffuse peritoneal carcinomatosis. Patients were treated with oxaliplatin-based HIPEC (460 mg/m^2) heated to 41.5°C for 30 min after cytoreductive surgery. This was followed by six more cycles of systemic IV infusion of oxaliplatin 100 mg/m^2 IV in combination with docetaxel 75 mg/m^2. Although there was no postoperative mortality, 28% of patients had major postoperative complications, most commonly hemorrhage (28%), followed by abdominal abscess (4%), sepsis (4%), and central vein thrombosis (4%). After a median follow-up of 18 months, the relapse rate was 28, and 96% of the patients were alive. The median disease free survival (DFS) was 10 months.

9.2.2
Floxuridine (FUDR)

Intraperitoneal administration of the fluoropyrimidine, FUDR, was studied at USC, NYU [15, 18, 19], and the Gastrointestinal Service at MSKCC [38]. The rationale for these studies was based on the theoretical advantages of this drug over 5-fluorouracil (Table 9.3) [18, 39–41]. Moreover, the Southwest Oncology Group (SWOG) randomized phase II study of IP mitoxantrone or FUDR selected FUDR as being promising for subsequent studies [42]. However, interest in this class of drugs for ovarian cancer treatment is low, and subsequent development has focused on applying it postoperatively in patients with locally advanced gastric cancer undergoing curative resections [43]. Nevertheless, phase I activity was seen among ovarian cancer patients treated for small volume recurrence with FUDR in combination with cisplatin, carboplatin, or both [44].

Table 9.3 Comparison of 5-fluorouracil (5FU) and floxuridine (FUDR) for IP administration

Feature	5FU	FUDR	Comment [reference]
Cytotoxicity in vitro (EC$_{50}$)	In 10–100 nanomolar range	Below 1 to nanomolar range	FUDR more cytotoxic [41]
Solubility	Insoluble in acid pH	No solubility problems	Favors FUDR [package inserts]
Peritoneal tolerance and complications	Pain during IP, fibrosis [39]	Only one report of fibrosis [40]	Unlikely with FUDR
Liver clearance	Extensive first-pass	Extensive first-pass	More complete with FUDR [18]
Other features of pharmacology	Catabolic products may be neurotoxic	FUDR gives rise to sustained 5FU concentrations	FUDR and 5FU: possible independent antitumor effects

9.2.3
Topotecan

Topotecan is a major drug for the treatment of recurrent ovarian cancer. While being active in the recurrent setting, it has not shown promise for short-term IV consolidation. The use of IP topotecan and other topoisomerase-I inhibitors [45–52] offer some theoretical benefits: (1) greater exposure to the active lactone form in the acid pH of the peritoneum; (2) pharmacologic advantage vis-à-vis the systemic route; and (3) improved therapeutic index, particularly with regard to myelosuppression, when combined with a platinum, both given at lower doses by the IP route. Results from a trial at NYU have confirmed these benefits [45]. Other reports have indicated a good therapeutic index and activity by the IP route, alone or in combination with other drugs [46, 48, 50–52]. A recent preclinical study shows significant enhancement of IP topotecan activity in combination with IV anti-VEGF therapy (see below section "Bevacizumab"). The increased uptake of topotecan into tumor nodules by diffusion when an agent such as bevacizumab is added supports future phase III studies of topotecan combination therapy.

9.2.4
Irinotecan

Preclinical data suggest that irinotecan, a toposomerase I inhibitor, has potential advantages when given by the IP route, [47, 53] which was supported by a recent phase I and pharmacologic study of this drug at USC (El-Khoueiry A, personal communication). Patients with mucinous tumors might derive special benefit, given the activity of this drug against colon cancer by the systemic route. A molecular profile of the high expression of thymidylate synthase and the presence of microsatellite instability predict for resistance to fluoropyrimidines and enhanced responsiveness to topoisomerase-I inhibitors [53]. Moreover, mucinous tumors are often characterized by a lesser propensity to invade, and to spread within the peritoneal cavity giving rise to large intraabdominal masses that displace and compress organs. These peritoneal surface malignances have been treated by hyperthermic perfusion as described by Sugarbaker in this text.

9.2.5
Gemcitabine

Gemcitabine, a pyrimidine base, has demonstrated antitumor activity against a number of solid tumors. It first gained U.S. Food and Drug Administration (FDA) approval in 1996 for the treatment of advanced pancreatic cancer. Several IV schedules of gemcitabine have been examined in phase I trials [54], but subsequent trials have primarily utilized the weekly schedule for pancreatic cancer [55]. A trial of IP administration of gemcitabine in pancreatic cancer was reported in 2004 [56]. Morgan et al. [17] conducted a phase I trial in which IP gemcitabine was given twice a week for 2 weeks during a 28-day cycle to 30 heavily pretreated patients with peritoneal carcinomatosis, 14 of whom had ovarian cancer. The achieved mean pharmacologic advantage ($AUC_{peritoneal}/AUC_{plasma}$) of more than 800 was similar to or better than that seen with other agents administered IP. Although there were no responses, three patients, including one with ovarian cancer, had their ascites controlled. In addition, the CA-125 tumor marker was reduced from 500 to 102 for an ovarian cancer patient in this trial. Dose-limiting toxicities were gastrointestinal, respiratory (including one fatal event), and elevation of alanine aminotransferase. Based on this study, the investigators recommended 120 mg/m^2 twice weekly for the phase II trial. Sabbatini et al. [57] carried out a gemcitabine and IP cisplatin phase I/II combination study; myelosuppression was the dose-limiting toxicity. Initially, IP cisplatin was given on day 1 at 75 mg/m^2 with gemcitabine at 500, 750, 1,000, or 1,250 mg/m^2 IP on days 1, 8, and 15 every 28-days for four courses. However, the phase I dose-limiting toxicity of grade 3 thrombocytopenia resulted in a protocol revision to reduce the gemcitabine dose. In phase II, 30 patients were given gemcitabine 500 mg/m^2 on days 1 and 8 in combination with IP cisplatin 75 mg/m^2 every 3 weeks for four courses. The median time to treatment failure and overall survival was 15.9 and 43.5 months, respectively [57]. This combination has not been examined further in clinical studies.

9.3
Other Methods to Potentiate IP Cisplatin

A *liposomal* preparation of cisplatin, c-SLIT, initially developed for aerosol administration to treat pulmonary metastases [58], has shown an improved therapeutic index when delivered IP to rodents in comparison to cisplatin. Clinical studies have been planned, but not yet carried out.

Cyclosporin has been known to enhance cisplatin and/or carboplatin action and may possibly overcome resistance [59]. Clinical studies have been performed by investigators at Yale, and some antitumor activity has been seen [60].

Bortezomib is capable of inhibiting the proteasome-mediated degradation of CTR1, a copper transporter that is also involved in the intracellular transport of cisplatin and carboplatin. Under conditions of such inhibition, additional amounts of cisplatin might be taken up intracellularly. Work in Howell's laboratory has been optimizing the conditions for possible synergy in preparation for a clinical study (described elsewhere in this text). Studies comparing IP cisplatin (used as consolidation) versus IP cisplatin plus bortezomib or other modulators are worth considering in patients who undergo surgical or clinical reassessments after initial induction.

9.4
Radioimmunotherapy

Treatment of ovarian cancer with IP radioimmunotherapy using β-emitter 90Y-HMFG1 failed to demonstrate improvement either in progression-free or overall survival in a phase III trial [61]. Andersson et al. [62] hypothesized that the use of α-emitter would be more advantageous because of the following: shorter half-line and less bone marrow irradiation; short range and heavier α-particles may be more effective for the elimination of small tumor cell aggregates; heavier α-particles transfer higher energy better than much lighter β-particles. Preclinical studies with α-emitter 211At-MX F(ab9)$_2$ have shown therapeutic efficacy in a mouse model of ovarian carcinoma [63].

In a phase I study, nine patients with relapsed ovarian cancer in complete remission after salvage chemotherapy confirmed by laparoscopy underwent IP treatment with 211At α-emitter labeled to MX35 F(ab9)$_2$ using the compound N-succinimidyl-3-(trimethylstannyl)-benzoate [62]. The investigators reported no adverse effects. After median follow-up of 23 months, three of nine patients remained in clinical remission, CA-125 elevation was detected in five patients, and only one patient had died from ovarian cancer [62].

9.5
Immune Modulation and Antibodies

T-cells and macrophages are abundant in the peritoneal cavity of patients with ovarian cancer [64, 65]. T-cells derived from patients with ovarian cancer secrete tumor necrosis factor alpha (TNF-α) and interferon gamma (IFN-γ) in both an antigen-independent and an antigen-dependent fashion [66]. Moreover, T-cell lines derived from patients with ovarian cancer demonstrate antitumor activity in the setting of low-dose recombinant IL-2 [67–69]. Vaccines and Bacillus Calmette-Guérin (BCG) were the first IP therapies to demonstrate response [70]. These agents were followed by cytokines, such as recombinant IFNs, and interleukins. The advantages of cytokines for IP therapy include: large molecular size and long duration of stay in the peritoneal cavity; cytokine pharmacokinetics theoretically achieving a higher mean pharmacologic advantage ($AUC_{peritoneal}/AUC_{plasma}$) than with chemotherapeutic agents; and main drainage through lymphatics rather than blood, theoretically stimulating T-cells along the way and killing regional lymph node-based metastases [71].

Alpha-interferon (α-IFN) was initially studied as a single-agent and then in combination with cisplatin in the setting of minimal residual disease. The GOG 0102 series clearly delineated what might be required in order to experience some benefit (Table 9.2). IFN-γ, TNF-α, and other specific immunostimulation therapies have been used to treat ovarian cancer via the IP route. This subject was thoroughly reviewed in 2000 [72]. Additional studies using immune modulation, including gene-therapy mediated restoration of tumor suppressor genes and immunotoxins against T-regulatory cells are on going [73].

Interleukin-2 triggers CD4+ T-cell differentiation from T-cell precursors. In addition, IL-2 promotes CD4+ T-cell expansion, mediates activation of natural killer (NK) cells and CD8+ T-cells including CD8+ memory T-cells [74, 75]. Studies conducted at the NCI were among the first to study IP IL-2 [76]. NCI investigators studied the effects of IL-2 and lymphokine-activated killer (LAK) cells in both murine models and in clinical trials [77]. Recently, interest in IL-2 has been revitalized based on an updated analysis of the long-term survival in ovarian cancer. Two trials [78, 79] were conducted using IP injections of IL-2 in patients with ovarian cancer. In the first trial, 45 very heavily pretreated patients with ovarian cancer (six or more courses of prior platinum-based chemotherapy) and laparotomy-confirmed active ovarian cancer were enrolled to receive either intermittent weekly

24-h infusions or continuous 7-day infusions followed by 7-day intervals without treatment. Locoregional dose-limiting toxicities with the 7-day infusion schedule were bowel perforation and hypotension at a dose of 600,000 IU/m^2 (the maximum tolerated dose, or MTD, of IL-2). Among the 35 evaluable patients, the response rate was 25.7% (17% laparotomy-confirmed complete response, 8% partial response). The reported median survival time was 13.7 months with the overall 5-year survival probability of 13.9%. For the nine responding patients, the median survival time had not been reached by the time of publication (range, 27 to more than 90 months) [78]. In the second, open label phase II trial by the same investigators, 31 very heavily pretreated (six or more prior courses of therapy) patients with ovarian cancer were given recombinant IL-2 at a dose of 600,000 IU/m^2 weekly for 16 weeks. Remarkably, among the 24 evaluable patients, the overall response was 25% and complete response was 17%. Median survival was 25.2 months. For the four patients with complete response, the mean time to disease progression was 22.5 months (range, 4–54 months). The reason why IL-2 produces response rates around 10–20% among many of human tumors is unknown. CD4+CD25+FOXP3+ regulatory T (Treg) cells likely mediate tumor cell evasion of the human immune system. IL-2-stimulated proliferation of Treg cells potentially blunts its own stimulation of the host immune system [79]. Recently, *IL-2 conjugated with diphtheria toxin* has been administered IP to ovarian cancer patients in order to eliminate Treg cells, as a way of inducing a favorable antitumor immunity (protocol at the University of Washington, ML Disis, study chair).

Interleukin-12 (IL-12) is a large cytokine with a theoretically longer residence time when given by the IP route [72]. IL-12 triggers production of IFN-γ and TNF-α. It mediates activation and action of NK cells, LAK cells, and cytotoxic T-cells. It has also been shown to inhibit angiogenesis [80]. Lenzi et al. [81] conducted a phase II multiinstitutional trial of IP IL-12 in patients with ovarian and primary peritoneal carcinoma. There were no responses but two patients with stable disease were available among 12 patients, that had response assessment. Grade 3 fatigue (four patients) and grade 4 neutropenia (one patient) were the main toxicities [81].

Trastuzumab, pertuzumab (2C4), and their immunotoxin derivatives merit consideration for IP administration, given the increased expression of Her2 in the presence of progressive involvement of the peritoneum by ovarian cancer [82]. Several studies have failed to show any prognostic significance to Her2 expression and an inconsistent relationship with histologic subtypes. Nevertheless, interest in revisiting this area is spurred by the recent positive trial of systemic trastuzumab in gastric cancer when added to chemotherapy [83], and interest in immunoconjugates.

9.6
Bevacizumab

Bevacizumab is discussed as a part of standard IP regimens covered by Alberts (Chapter 4 in this volume); pilot studies adding IV bevacizumab to IP cisplatin and paclitaxel have reported the feasibility of inhibiting angiogenesis while delivering IP therapy. Preclinical models of ovarian cancer have studied the depth of penetration of IP administered doxorubicin

[3]. More recently, the ability of antiangiogenic drugs to achieve a reduction in tumor vessel permeability, density, and diameter [84, 85] make them a potential option as adjunct agents to IP chemotherapy [86]. Shah et al. [86] studied bevacizumab in combination with IP or systemic topotecan, and in combination with IP or systemic cisplatin in the A2780 human xenograft model of ovarian carcinoma. Bevacizumab enhanced the concentrations of topotecan or cisplatin when administered by the IP route. This resulted in a better outcome for the mice treated IP over those treated with either systemic topotecan or cisplatin with bevacizumab. The striking effects of altering tumor angiogenesis on intratumoral drug concentrations following IP administration are further covered by Howell elsewhere in this text. Furthermore, these experiments are a powerful rationale behind a new phase III clinical trial by the GOG (GOG 0252, which began enrollment in August 2009) comparing IP versus IV drug administration, both with bevacizumab, in the first-line treatment of ovarian cancer.

9.7
Discussion

The approaches listed above provide the foundation for eventual testing of new IP agents in phase III studies. The addition of bevacizumab to standard first-line IP approaches represents the first logical phase III trial. IP drug delivery may have advantages over systemic administration, although with continued caveats related to logistics and patient tolerance. Several of the chemotherapeutic agents listed should be evaluated in circumstances not currently studied by cooperative groups. For example, IP consolidation should prove informative for topotecan in combination with cisplatin. A positive result would be indicative of superiority of IP vs. systemic effects for topotecan, since several phase III studies with IV consolidation of topotecan have been negative. Phase I/II studies are also justified in patients with small volume disease at reassessment. Contrary to the experience two decades ago, translational studies accompanying the evaluation of new drugs may now be more effectively applied. In particular, antibodies and liposomal preparations may be delivered by the IP route in smaller amounts while leading enhanced therapeutic effects. Apart from the studies in front-line ovarian cancer, it is imperative to explore these novel agents in a range of clinical circumstances.

References

1. Dedrick RL, Myers CE, Bungay PM, DeVita VT Jr (1978) Pharmacokinetic rationale for peritoneal administration in the treatment of ovarian cancer. Cancer Treat Rep 62:1–11
2. Jones RB, Collins JM, Myers CE et al (1981) High-volume intraperitoneal chemotherapy with methotrexate in patients with cancer. Cancer Res 41:55–59
3. Ozols R, Locker GY, Doroshow JH, Grotzinger KR, Myers CE, Young RC (1979) Pharmacokinetics of adriamycin and tissue penetration in murine ovarian cancer. Cancer Res 39: 3209–3214
4. Ozols RF, Young RC, Speyer JL, Sugarbaker PH, Greene R, Jenkins J, Myers CE (1982) Phase I and pharmacological studies of adriamycin administered intraperitoneally to patients with ovarian cancer. Cancer Res 42:4265–4269

5. Speyer JL, Collins JM, Dedrick RL et al (1980) Phase I and pharmacological studies of 5-fluoruracil administered intraperitoneally. Cancer Res 40:567–572
6. Speyer JL, Sugarbaker PH, Collins JM, Dedrick RL, Klecker RW Jr, Myers CE (1981) Portal levels and hepatic clearance of 5-fluorouracil after intraperitoneal administration in humans. Cancer Res 41:1916–1922
7. Sugarbaker PH, Gianola FJ, Speyer JL, Wesley R, Barofsky I, Myers CE (1985) Prospective, randomized trial of intravenous versus intraperitoneal 5-fluorouracil in patients with advanced primary colon or rectal cancer. Semin Oncol 12(3 suppl 4):101–111
8. Elias D, Bonnay M, Puizillou JM et al (2002) Heated intra-operative intraperitoneal oxaliplatin after complete resection of peritoneal carcinomatosis: pharmacokinetics and tissue distribution. Ann Oncol 13:267–272
9. Howell SB, Pfeiffle CE, Wung WE, Olshen RA (1983) Intraperitoneal cis-diamminedichloroplatinum with systemic thiosulfate protection. Cancer Res 43:1426–1431
10. Howell SB, Pfeiffle CL, Wung WE et al (1982) Intraperitoneal cisplatin with systemic thiosulfate protection. Ann Intern Med 97:845–851
11. Speyer JL, Beller U, Colombo N et al (1990) Intraperitoneal carboplatin: favorable results in women with minimal residual ovarian cancer after cisplatin therapy. J Clin Oncol 8:1335–1341
12. Feun LG, Blessing JA, Major FJ, DiSaia PJ, Alvarez RD, Berek JS (1998) A Phase II study of intraperitoneal cisplatin and thiotepa in residual ovarian carcinoma: a Gynecologic Oncology Group study. Gynecol Oncol 7(3):410–415
13. Howell SB, Pfeifle CE, Olshen RA (1984) Intraperitoneal chemotherapy with melphalan. Ann Intern Med 101(1):14–18
14. Sugarbaker PH, Stuart OA, Carmignani CP (2006) Pharmacokinetic changes induced by the volume of chemotherapy solution in patients treated with hyperthermic intraperitoneal mitomycin C. Cancer Chemother Pharmacol 57:703–708
15. Israel VK, Jiang C, Muggia FM et al (1995) Intraperitoneal 5-fluoro-2'deoxyuridine (FUDR) and (S)-leucovorin for disease predominantly confined to the peritoneal cavity: a pharmacokinetic and toxicity study. Cancer Chemother Pharmacol 37(1–2):32–38
16. King ME, Pfeiffle CE, Howell SB (1984) Intraperitoneal cytosine arabinoside therapy in ovarian carcinoma. J Clin Oncol 2(6):662–699
17. Morgan RJ Jr, Synold TW, Xi B, Lim D, Shibata S, Margolin K, Schwarz RE, Leong L, Somolo G, Twadorski P, Yen Y, Chow W, Tetef M, Lin P, Paz B, Kocywas M, Wagman L, Chu D, Frankel P, Stalter S, Doroshow JH (2007) Phaase I trial of intraperitoneal gemcitabine in the treatment of advanced malignancies primarily confined to the peritoneal cavity. Clin Cancer Res 13:1232–1237
18. Muggia FM, Chan KK, Russell C et al (1991) Phase I and pharmacologic evaluation of intraperitoneal 5-fluoro-2'-deoxyuridine. Cancer Chemother Pharmacol 28(4):241–250
19. Muggia FM, Tulpule A, Retzios A et al (1994) Intraperitoneal 5-fluoro-2'-deoxyuridine with escalating doses of leucovorin: pharmacology and clinical tolerance. Invest New Drugs 12(3):197–206
20. Markman M, Rowinsky E, Hakes T et al (1992) Phase I trial of intraperitoneal taxol: a Gynecologic Oncology Group study. J Clin Oncol 10(9):1485–1491
21. Morgan RJ Jr, Doroshow JH, Synold T, Lim D, Shibata S, Margolin K, Schwartz R, Leong L, Somio G, Twardowski P, Yen Y, Chow W, Lin P, Paz B, Chu D, Frankel P, Stalter S (2003) Phase I trial of intraperitoneal docetaxel in the treatment of advanced malignancies primarily confined to the peritoneal cavity: dose-limiting toxicity and pharmacokinetics. Clin Cancer Res 9(16 pt 1):5896–5901
22. Alberts DS, Markman M, Muggia F, Ozols RF, Eldermire E, Bookman MA, Chen T, Curtin J, Hess LM, Liebes L, Young RC, Trimble E (2006) Proceedings of a GOG workshop on intraperitoneal therapy for ovarian cancer. Gynecol Oncol 103(3):783–792
23. Howell SB, Kirmani S, Lucas WE et al (1990) A phase II trial of intraperitoneal cisplatin and etoposide for primary treatment of ovarian epithelial cancer. J Clin Oncol 8(1):137–145

24. O'Dwyer PJ, LaCreta FP, Daugherty JP, Hogan M, Rosenblum NG, O'Dwyer JL, Comis RL (1991) Phase I pharmacokinetic study of intraperitoneal etoposide. Cancer Res 51(8): 2041–2046

25. Muggia FM, Groshen S, Russell C, Jeffers S, Chen SC, Schlaerth J, Curtin J, Morrow CP (1993) Intraperitoneal carboplatin and etoposide for persistent epithelial ovarian cancer after platinum-based regimens. Gynecol Oncol 50(2):232–238

26. Piver MS, Lele SB, Marchetti DL, Baker TR, Emrich LJ, Hartman AB (1988) Surgically documented response to intraperitoneal cisplatin, cytarabine, and bleomycin after intravenous cisplatin-based chemotherapy in advanced ovarian adenocarcinoma. J Clin Oncol 6(11):1679–1684

27. Reichman B, Markman M, Hakes T et al (1989) Intraperitoneal cisplatin and etoposide in the treatment of refractory/recurrent ovarian carcinoma. J Clin Oncol 7:1327–1332

28. Berek JS, Markman M, Blessing JA, Kucera PR, Nelson BE, Anderson B, Hanjani P (1999) Intraperitoneal alpha-interferon alternating with cisplatin in residual ovarian carcinoma: a Phase II Gynecologic Oncology Group study. Gynecol Oncol 74(1):48–52

29. Berek JS, Markman M, Stonebraker B, Lentz SS, Adelson MD, DeGeest K, Moore D (1999) Intraperitoneal interferon-alpha in residual ovarian carcinoma: a Phase II Gynecologic Oncology Group study. Gynecol Oncol 75(1):10–14

30. Braly PS, Berek JS, Blessing JA, Homesley HD, Averette H (1995) Intraperitoneal administration of cisplatin and 5-fluorouracil in residual ovarian cancer: a Phase II Gynecologic Oncology Group trial. Gynecol Oncol 56(2):164–168

31. Markman M, Berek JS, Blessing JA, McGuire WP, Bell J, Homesley HD (1992) Characteristics of patients with small-volume residual ovarian cancer unresponsive to cisplatin-based IP chemotherapy: lessons learned from a Gynecologic Oncology Group phase II trial of IP cisplatin and recombinant alpha-interferon. Gynecol Oncol 45(1):3–8

32. Markman M, Blessing JA, Major F, Manetta A (1993) Salvage intraperitoneal therapy of ovarian cancer employing cisplatin and etoposide: a Gynecologic Oncology Group study. Gynecol Oncol 50(2):191–195

33. Markman M, Reichman B, Hakes T et al (1993) Evidence supporting the superiority of intraperitoneal cisplatin compared to intraperitoneal carboplatin for salvage therapy of small-volume residual ovarian cancer. Gynecol Oncol 50(1):100–104

34. Fujiwara K, Suzuki S, Ishikawa H et al (2005) Preliminary toxicity analysis of intraperitoneal carboplatin in combination with intravenous paclitaxel chemotherapy for patients with carcinoma of the ovary, peritoneum, or fallopian tube. Int J Gynaecol Oncol 3:426–431

35. Ferron G, Gesson-Paute A, Gladieff L, Thomas F, Chatelut E, Querleu D et al (2009) Laparoscopically assisted heated intra-operative chemotherapy (HIPEC): technical aspect and pharmacokinetics data. In: Bonetti A et al (eds) Platinum and other heavy metal compounds in cancer chemotherapy. Humana Press, New York, pp 343–351

36. Elias D, Lefevre JH, Chevalier J, Brouquet A, Marchal F, Classe JM, Ferron G, Guilloit JM, Meeus P, Goéré D, Bonastre J (2009) Complete cytoreductive surgery plus intraperitoneal chemohyperthermia with oxaliplatin for peritoneal carcinomatosis of colorectal origin. J Clin Oncol 27(5):681–685

37. Fagotti A, Paris I, Grimolizzi F, Fanfani F, Vizzielli G, Naldini A, Scambia G (2009) Secondary cytoreduction plus oxaliplatin-based HIPEC in platinum-sensitive recurrent ovarian cancer patients: a pilot study. Gynecol Oncol 113(3):335–340

38. Brenner B, Shah MA, Karpeh MS, Gonen M, Brennan MF, Coit DG, Klimstra DS, Tang LH, Kelsen DP (2006) A phase II trial of neoadjuvant cisplatin–fluorouracil followed by postoperative intraperitoneal floxuridine–leucovorin in patients with locally advanced gastric cancer. Ann Oncol 17(9):1404–1411

39. Atiq OT, Kelsen DP, Shiu MH, Saltz L, Tong W, Niedzwiecki D, Trochanowski B, Lin S, Toomasi F, Brennan M (1993) Phase II trial of postoperative adjuvant intraperitoneal cisplatin and fluorouracil and systemic fluorouracil chemotherapy in patients with resected gastric cancer. J Clin Oncol 11:425–433

40. Fata F, Ron IG, Maluf F, Klimstra D, Kemeny N (2000) Intra-abdominal fibrosis after systemic and intraperitoneal therapy containing fluoropyrimidines. Cancer 88:2447–2451
41. Park JG, Collins JM, Gazdar AF, Allegra CJ, Steinberg SM, Greene RF, Kramer BS (1988) Enhancement of fluorinated pyrimidine-induced cytotoxicity by leucovorin in human colorectal carcinoma cell lines. J Natl Cancer Inst 80:1560–1564
42. Muggia FM, Liu PY, Alberts DS, Wallace DL, O'Toole RV, Terada KY, Franklin EW, Herrer GW, Goldberg DA, Hannigan EV (1996) Intraperitoneal mitoxantrone or floxuridine: effects on time-to-failure and survival in patients with minimal residual ovarian cancer after second-look laparotomy – a randomized phase II study by the Southwest Oncology Group. Gynecol Oncol 61:395–402
43. Newman E, Potmesil M, Ryan T, Marcus S, Hiotis S, Yee H, Norwood B, Wendell M, Muggia F, Hochster H (2005) Neoadjuvant chemotherapy, surgery and adjuvant intraperitoneal chemotherapy in patients with locally advanced gastric or gastroesophageal junction carcinoma: a phase II study. Semin Oncol 32:S97–S100
44. Muggia FM, Jeffers S, Muderspach L et al (1997) Phase I/II study of intraperitoneal floxuridine and platinums (cisplatin and/or carboplatin). Gynecol Oncol 66:290–294
45. Andreopoulou E, Chen T, Liebes L, Lu J, Moore S, Fusco E, Liu P, Curtin J, Hochster H, Muggia F (2005) Phase I/pharmacology study of intraperitoneal (IP) 3–5 day topotecan alone and with cisplatin on day 1: potential for consolidation in ovarian cancer. ASCO Meet Abstr 23:5045
46. Bos AM, De Vos FY, de Vries EG, Beijnen JH, Rosing H, Mourits MJ, van der Zee AG, Gietema JA, Willemse PH (2005) A phase I study of intraperitoneal topotecan in combination with intravenous carboplatin and paclitaxel in advanced ovarian cancer. Eur J Cancer 41:539–548
47. Choi SH, Tsuchida Y, Yang HW (1998) Oral versus intraperitoneal administration of irinotecan in the treatment of human neuroblastoma in nude mice. Cancer Lett 124:15–21
48. Hofstra LS, Bos AM, de Vries EG, van der Zee AG, Beijnen JH, Rosing H, Mulder NH, Aalders JG, Willemse PH (2001) A phase I and pharmacokinetic study of intraperitoneal topotecan. Br J Cancer 85:1627–1633
49. Muggia F, Liebes L, Potmesil M, Hamilton A, Hochster H, Hornreich G, Sorich J, Downey A, Wasserstrom H (2000) Intraperitoneal topoisomerase-I inhibitors: preliminary findings with 9-aminocamptothecin. Ann N Y Acad Sci 922:178–187
50. Muntz HG, Malpass TW, McGonigle KF, Robertson MD, Weiden PL (2008) Phase II study of intraperitoneal topotecan as consolidation chemotherapy in ovarian cancer. Cancer 113(3): 490–496
51. Plaxe SC, Christen RD, O'Quigley J, Braly PS, Freddo JL, McClay E, Heath D, Howell SB (1998) Phase I and pharmacokinetic study of intraperitoneal topotecan. Invest New Drugs 16: 147–153
52. Sood AK, Lush R, Geisler JP, Shahin MS, Sanders L, Sullivan D, Buller RE, Sorosky JI (2004) Sequential intraperitoneal topotecan and oral etoposide chemotherapy in recurrent platinum-resistant ovarian carcinoma: results of a phase II trial. Clin Cancer Res 10:6080–6085
53. Elias D, Goere D, Blot F, Billard V, Pocard M, Kohneh-Shahri N, Raynard B (2007) Optimization of hyperthermic intraperitoneal chemotherapy with oxaliplatin plus irinotecan at 43°C after complete cytoreductive surgery: mortality and morbidity in 106 consecutive patients. Ann Surg Oncol 14:1818–1824
54. Hertel LW, Boder GB, Kroin JS, Rinzel SM, Poore GA, Todd GC, Grindey GB (1990) Evaluation of the antitumor activity of gemcitabine (2′, 2′-difluoro-2′-deoxycytidine). Cancer Res 50:4417–4422
55. Burris HA III, Moore MJ, Andersen J, Green MR, Rothenberg ML, Modiano MR, Cripps MC, Von Hoff DD (1997) Improvements in survival and clinical benefit with gemcitabine as first-line therapy for patients with advanced pancreas cancer: a randomized trial. J Clin Oncol 15(6):2403–2413

56. Gamblin TC, Egorin MJ, Zuhowski EG, Lagattuta TF, Herscher LL, Russo A, Libutti SK, Alexander HR, Dedrick RL, Bartlett DL (2004) Intraperitoneal gemcitabine therapy for advanced adenocarcinoma of the pancreas. Ann Surg Oncol 11(suppl 2):S55

57. Sabbatini P, Aghajanian C, Leitao M, Venkatraman E, Anderson S, Dupont J, Dizon D, O'Flaherty C, Bloss J, Chi D, Spriggs D (2004) Intraperitoneal cisplatin with intraperitoneal gemcitabine in patients with epithelial ovarian cancer: results of a phase I/II Trial. Clin Cancer Res 10:2962–2967

58. Wittgen BP, Kunst PW, van der Born K, van Wijk AW, Perkins W, Pilkiewicz FG, Perez-Soler R, Nicholson S, Peters GJ, Postmus PE (2007) Phase I study of aerosolized SLIT cisplatin in the treatment of patients with carcinoma of the lung. Clin Cancer Res 13(8):2414–2421

59. Morgan RJ Jr, Synold TW, Gandara D, Muggia F, Scudder S, Reed E, Margolin K, Raschko J, Leong L, Shibata S, Tetef M, Vasilev S, McGonigle K, Longmate J, Yen Y, Chow W, Somlo G, Carroll M, Doroshow JH (2004) Phase II trial of carboplatin and infusional cyclosporine in platinum-resistant recurrent ovarian cancer. Cancer Chemother Pharmacol 54(4):283–289

60. Chambers SK, Chambers JT, Davis CA, Kohorn EI, Schwartz PE, Lorber MI, Handschumacher RE, Pizzorno G (1997) Pharmacokinetic and phase I trial of intraperitoneal carboplatin and cyclosporine in refractory ovarian cancer patients. J Clin Oncol 15:1945–1952

61. Verheijen RH, Massuger LF, Benigno BB, Epenetos AA, Lopes A, Soper JT, Markowska J, Vyzula R, Jobling T, Stamp G, Spiegel G, Thurston D, Falke T, Lambert J, Seiden MV (2006) Phase III trial of intraperitoneal therapy with yttrium-90-labeled HMFG1 murine monoclonal antibody in patients with epithelial ovarian cancer after a surgically defined complete remission. J Clin Oncol 24:571–578

62. Andersson H, Cederkrantz E, Bäck T, Divgi C, Elgqvist J, Himmelman J, Horvath G, Jacobsson L, Jensen H, Lindegren S, Palm S, Hultborn R (2009) Intraperitoneal alpha-particle radioimmunotherapy of ovarian cancer patients: pharmacokinetics and dosimetry of 211At-MX35 F(ab9)2 – a phase I study. J Nucl Med 50:1153–1160

63. Palm S, Bäck T, Claesson I, Danielsson A, Elgqvist J, Frost S, Hultborn R, Jensen H, Lindegren S, Jacobsson L (2007) Therapeutic efficacy of astatine-211-labeled trastuzumab on radioresistant SKOV-3 tumors in nude mice. Int J Radiat Oncol Biol Phys 69:572–579

64. Freedman RS, Kudelka AP, Kavanagh JJ, Verschraegen C, Edwards CL, Nash M, Levy L, Atkinson EN, Zhang HZ, Melichar B, Patenia R, Templin S, Scott W, Platsoucas CD (2000) Clinical and biologic effects of intraperitoneal injections of recombinant interferon-γ, and recombinant interleukin-2 with or without tumor infiltrating lymphocytes in patients with ovarian or peritoneal carcinoma. Clin Cancer Res 6:2268–2278

65. Melichar B, Tousková M, Tosner J, Kopecký O (2001) The phenotype of ascitic fluid lymphocytes in patients with ovarian carcinoma and other primaries. Onkologie 24:156–160

66. Kooi S, Freedman RS, Rodriguez-Villanueva J, Platsoucas CD (1993) Cytokine production by T-cell lines derived from tumor-infiltrating lymphocytes (TIL) from patients with ovarian carcinoma: tumor-specific immune responses and inhibition of antigen-independent cytokine production by ovarian tumor cells. Lymphokine Cytokine Res 12:429–437

67. Freedman RS, Tomasovic B, Templin S, Atkinson EN, Kudelka A, Edwards CL, Platsoucas CD (1994) Large-scale expansion in interleukin-2 of tumor-infiltrating lymphocytes from patients with ovarian carcinoma for adoptive immunotherapy. J Immunol Methods 167:145–160

68. Ioannides CG, Freedman RS, Platsoucas CD, Rashed S, Kim YP (1991) Cytotoxic T cell clones isolated from ovarian tumor-infiltrating lymphocytes recognize multiple antigenic epitopes on autologous tumor cells. J Immunol 146:1700–1707

69. Ioannides CG, Platsoucas CD, Rashed S, Wharton JT, Edwards CL, Freedman RS (1991) Tumor cytolysis by lymphocytes infiltrating ovarian malignant ascites. Cancer Res 51:4257–4265

70. Freedman RS (1985) Recent immunologic advances affecting the management of ovarian cancer. In: Quillan EJ, Wharton JT (eds) Clinical obstetrics and gynecology, vol 28. Harper and Row, Philadelphia, pp 849–867

71. Hwu P, Freedman RS (2002) The immunotherapy of patients with ovarian cancer. J Immunother 25(3):189–201
72. Elkas JC, Dorigo O, Berek JS (2000) Intraperitoneal biologic therapy for ovarian cancer. In: Markman M (ed) Regional cancer therapy. Humana Press, New York, pp 193–211
73. Adams SF, Levine DA, Cadungog MG, Hammond R, Facciabene A, Olvera N, Rubin SC, Boyd J, Gimotty PA, Coukos G (2009) Intraepithelial T cells and tumor proliferation: impact on the benefit from surgical cytoreduction in advanced serous ovarian cancer. Cancer 115:2891–2902
74. Paredes R, de Quiros JC Lopez Benaldo, Fernandez-Cruz E, Clotet B, Lane HC (2002) The potential role of interleukin-2 in patients with HIV infection. AIDS Rev 4:36–40
75. Williams MA, Tyznik AJ, Bevan MJ (2006) Interleukin-2 signals during priming are required for secondary expansion of CD8+ memory T cells. Nature 441:890–893
76. Lotze MT, Custer MC, Rosenberg SA (1986) Intraperitoneal administration of interleukin-2 in patients with cancer. Arch Surg 121(12):1373–1379
77. Ottow RT, Steller EP, Sugarbaker PH, Wesley RA, Rosenberg SA (1987) Immunotherapy of intraperitoneal cancer with interleukin 2 and lymphokine-activated killer cells reduces tumor load and prolongs survival in murine models. Cell Immunol 104:366–376
78. Edwards RP, Gooding W, Lembersky BC, Colonello K, Hammond R, Paradise C, Kowal CD, Kunschner AJ, Baldisseri M, Kirkwood JM, Herberman RB (1997) Comparison of toxicity and survival following intraperitoneal recombinant interleukin-2 for persistent ovarian cancer after platinum: twenty-four-hour versus 7-day infusion. J Clin Oncol 15:3399–3407
79. Wei S, Kryczek I, Edwards RP, Zou L, Szeliga W, Banerjee M, Cost M, Cheng P, Chang A, Redman B, Herberman RB, Zou W (2007) Interleukin-2 administration alters the CD4+FOXP3+ T-cell pool and tumor trafficking in patients with ovarian carcinoma. Cancer Res 67:7487–7494
80. Voest EE, Kenyon BM, O'Reilly MS, Truitt G, D'Amato RJ, Folkman J (1995) Inhibition of angiogenesis in vivo by interleukin-12. J Natl Cancer Inst 87:581–586
81. Lenzi R, Edwards R, June C, Seiden MV, Garcia ME, Rosenblum M, Freedman RS (2007) Phase II study of intraperitoneal recombinant interleukin-12 (rhIL-12) in patients with peritoneal carcinomatosis (residual disease < 1 cm) associated with ovarian cancer or primary peritoneal carcinoma. J Transl Med 5:66
82. Hellström I, Goodman G, Pullman J, Yang Y, Hellström KE (2001) Overexpression of HER-2 in ovarian carcinomas. Cancer Res 61(6):2420–2423
83. Van Cutsem E, Kang Y, Chung H, et al (2009) Efficacy results from the ToGA trial: a phase III study of trastuzumab added to standard chemotherapy (CT) in first-line human epidermal growth factor receptor 2 (HER2)-positive advanced gastric cancer (GC). J Clin Oncol 27(18 suppl):abstr LBA4509
84. Hu L, Hofmann J, Zaloudek C, Ferrara N, Hamilton T, Jaffe RB (2002) Vascular endothelial growth factor immunoneutralization plus paclitaxel markedly reduces tumor burden and ascites in athymic mouse model of ovarian cancer. Am J Pathol 161:1917–1924
85. Jain RK (2001) Normalizing tumor vasculature with anti-angiogenic therapy: a new paradigm for combination therapy. Nat Med 7:987–989
86. Shah DK, Shin BS, Veith J, Tóth K, Bernacki RJ, Balthasar JP (2009) Use of an anti-vascular endothelial growth factor antibody in a pharmacokinetic strategy to increase the efficacy of intraperitoneal chemotherapy. J Pharmacol Exp Ther 329:580–591
87. Alberts DS, Surwit EA, Peng YM, McCloskey T, Rivest R, Graham V, McDonald L, Roe D (1988) Phase I clinical and pharmacokinetic study of mitoxantrone given to patients by intraperitoneal administration. Cancer Res 48(20):5874–5877

Cytoreductive Surgery and Perioperative Intraperitoneal Chemotherapy: An Ongoing Research Effort

10

Paul H. Sugarbaker

10.1
Introduction

Ovarian cancer is the number one killer among gynecological malignancies. Information from the Surveillance, Epidemiology and End Results (SEER) program of the National Cancer Institute (NCI) shows that the incidence of ovarian cancer in the United States (U.S.) for all races has fluctuated between 14 and 16 per 100,000 persons during the 1991–2001 decade, and remains unchanged [1]. According to the same source, the U.S. estimated that complete prevalence was 167,002 women in 2001 [2]. Also, a woman living in the U.S. has a 0.117% probability of developing ovarian cancer until age 45 and a 1% probability of ovarian cancer until age 75 [3]. Ovarian cancer is the fifth most common cause of cancer death in Western countries [4].

Unfortunately, symptoms of ovarian cancer are unspecific and the diagnosis is rarely made early. A recent case-control study showed that when either increasing abdominal size, bloating, urinary urgency or pelvic pain occur more frequently, and with more intensity than expected or these symptoms are of recent onset, further investigation searching for an ovarian mass is warranted [5]. In the past, CA-125 tumor marker levels, transvaginal ultrasound, and pelvic examinations were thought to be potential effective screening tools. However, none of them have yet proved to decrease mortality from ovarian cancer [6]. Also, false positive tests lead to unnecessary emotional distress and invasive diagnostic procedures. As a consequence of its internal location and nonspecific symptomatology, most patients are diagnosed with ovarian cancer in late stages of the disease.

Most tumors are epithelial in origin (approximately 90%) and a minority are other histologic types. Once a tumor starts growing in the ovary, spread of cancer cells throughout the abdominopelvic cavity occurs very early in the natural history of the disease. Even a small primary cancer can rupture through the very thin ovarian capsule. The ovary is covered only by a thin layer of visceral peritoneum, easily disrupted by the expansion and the

P.H. Sugarbaker
Program in Peritoneal Surface Malignancy, Washington Cancer Institute,
106 Irving Street, NW, Suite 3900, Washington, DC, 20010, USA
e-mail: paul.sugarbaker@medstar.net

D.S. Alberts et al. (eds.), *Intraperitoneal Therapy for Ovarian Cancer*,
DOI: 10.1007/978-3-642-12130-2_10, © Springer-Verlag Berlin Heidelberg 2010

invasive nature of the cancerous growth. This early intracoelomic dissemination causes ovarian cancer to be a disease that is spread beyond the primary cancer site at the time of diagnosis [7, 8]. However, widespread peritoneal implantation is not the only route of dissemination. Depending on the stage of diagnosis, up to 50% of the women with ovarian cancer have pelvic or paraaortic lymph node involvement [9]. A smaller percentage of these women may develop hematogenous metastases in the liver, lungs, bone marrow, or brain.

In many patients, the natural history of ovarian cancer is similar to a gastrointestinal cancer with peritoneal surface dissemination. For example, similar to gastric cancer with carcinomatosis, the late consequences of this route of cancer spread are debilitating ascites formation and intestinal obstruction. With full knowledge of the natural history of progressive disease the targets of the treatment should be both the peritoneal surface spread as well as the systemic metastases. There can be no doubt that complete eradication of the peritoneal surface component of this disease would provide a major contribution to the overall management of this disease. Comprehensive management using surgical cytoreduction to decrease the tumor load to a minimum and perioperative intraperitoneal and systemic chemotherapy to eliminate macroscopic disease on peritoneal surfaces has the potential to greatly improve quality of life and have an impact on survival in women with ovarian cancer.

10.2
A Comprehensive Approach for Ovarian Cancer Treatment

The Program in Peritoneal Surface Malignancy at the Washington Cancer Institute has extensive experience with a treatment strategy that combines surgery plus perioperative chemotherapy. Cytoreductive surgery, including peritonectomy procedures and visceral resections, has been used in an attempt to eradicate all visible disease from the abdomen and pelvis. Peritonectomies are performed on demand; that is, only when there is visible disease on the peritoneal surface, these membranes stripped by electrosurgical dissection. Also, visceral resections are carried out as needed to clear the abdominal cavity from visible ovarian cancer. Retroperitoneal and pelvic lymphadenectomy are performed to resect palpably involved lymph nodes but systematic lymphadenectomy is not utilized. After all resections have been completed and before any reconstructions are performed, heated intraoperative intraperitoneal chemotherapy (HIPEC) with cisplatin and doxorubicin is administered with the goal of destroying microscopic residual disease and thereby preventing cancer cell implantation. These local-regional effects are augmented by systemic ifosfamide chemotherapy. The heated intraperitoneal chemotherapy combined with simultaneous systemic chemotherapy is referred to as HIPEC plus. As a result of surgical trauma and visceral manipulation, extensive raw tissue surfaces are vulnerable for cancer cell adherence and subsequent progression. Chemotherapy in the operating room is supplemented with the administration of early postoperative intraperitoneal chemotherapy (EPIC). EPIC is the use of an additional intraperitoneal chemotherapeutic agent during the first 5 days of the postoperative period.

The intraperitoneal route for administration of chemotherapy has been shown to improve progression-free survival and overall survival as compared to a systemic route in ovarian cancer patients [10–12]. However, a significant contrast exists between this prior experience and the comprehensive management discussed in this chapter. The efficacy and the simplicity of intraperitoneal chemotherapy administration may be greatly augmented by a perioperative timing of the chemotherapy delivery.

10.3
Selection Criteria for a Comprehensive Treatment Plan

Cytoreductive surgery and perioperative chemotherapy represent a comprehensive strategy for treatment of ovarian malignancies, requiring a knowledgeable selection of patients, a strong commitment from the surgical team, and institutional support.

Selection of patients is based on two well-defined criteria: ability of the patient to survive an extensive surgical procedure with acceptable morbidity and mortality and no evidence of clinical situations that would result in a futile surgical procedure. Patients of advanced age, poor performance status, malnourished or with medical conditions that would decrease the likelihood of postoperative survival should not be included. Also, patients with systemic metastases, multiple sites of bowel obstruction, common bile duct obstruction or ureteral obstruction should not be submitted to this comprehensive treatment because of residual disease following a surgical best effort.

This procedure requires dedication from a surgeon who must have broad surgical knowledge, a thorough understanding of intraperitoneal chemotherapy, strong technical skills and the stamina to endure long procedures. Realizing that these interventions are extensive and thereby costly, institutional backing is important. Early in the effort, Institutional Review Board (IRB) approval for HIPEC is advised to protect the patients, the surgeons and the institution. An effort to educate other physicians involved in this treatment, as well as nurses and ancillary personnel, should be undertaken. Standardized orders for chemotherapy as part of a well defined clinical pathway are necessary to coordinate the actions of the clinical staff. The steep learning curve that characterizes this treatment strategy makes it essential to design a careful plan and to regularly critically evaluate all the steps involved [13].

10.4
Quantitative Prognostic Indicators

The three quantitative prognostic indicators necessary for patient selection in order to treat patients most likely to benefit are, the prior surgical score (PSS), the peritoneal cancer index (PCI), and the completeness of cytoreduction (CC) score [14].

A convenient diagram is used as a guide in determining the PSS and the PCI (Fig. 10.1). Two transverse planes and two sagittal planes are used to divide the abdomen into nine

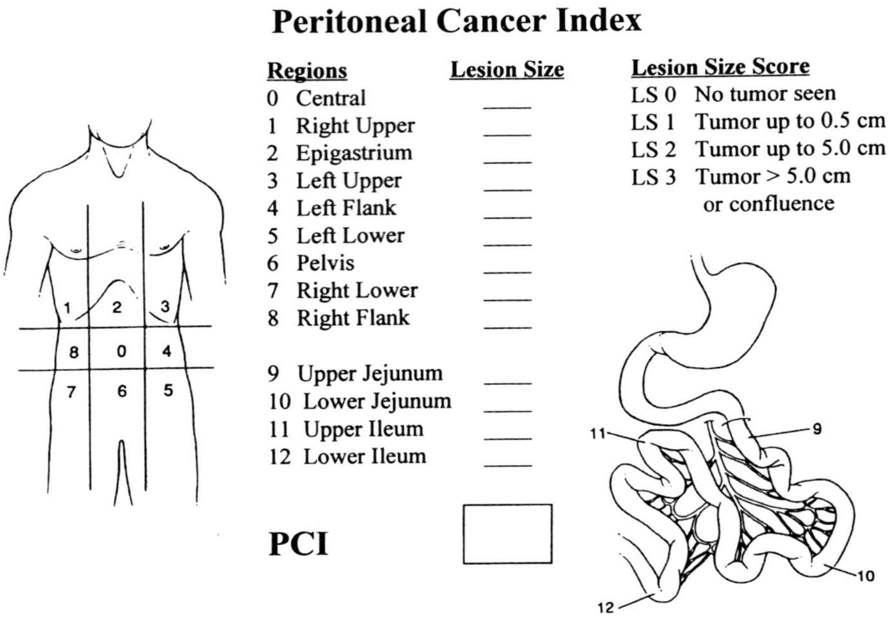

Peritoneal Cancer Index

Regions	Lesion Size	Lesion Size Score
0 Central	____	LS 0 No tumor seen
1 Right Upper	____	LS 1 Tumor up to 0.5 cm
2 Epigastrium	____	LS 2 Tumor up to 5.0 cm
3 Left Upper	____	LS 3 Tumor > 5.0 cm
4 Left Flank	____	or confluence
5 Left Lower	____	
6 Pelvis	____	
7 Right Lower	____	
8 Right Flank	____	
9 Upper Jejunum	____	
10 Lower Jejunum	____	
11 Upper Ileum	____	
12 Lower Ileum	____	

PCI

Fig. 10.1 Peritoneal cancer index (PCI)

abdominopelvic regions (AR). The upper transverse plane is located at the lowest aspect of the costal margin. The lower transverse plane is placed at the anterior superior iliac spine. The sagittal planes divide the abdomen into three equal sectors. These lines define nine AR, which are numbered in a clockwise direction with 0 at the umbilicus and 1 defining the space beneath the right hemidiaphragm. Regions 9 and 10 define the upper and lower portions of the jejunum, and regions 11 and 12 define the upper and lower portions of the ileum. The anatomic structures that are associated with each of these 13 regions have been designated [14].

Prior surgeries will modify the natural history of ovarian cancer by inducing cancer growth in crucial anatomic sites located beneath the peritoneal layer (along the ureters, in the groove between psoas muscle and vena cava, within the pelvic side wall). There can be no doubt that surgical trauma promotes cancer cell implantation and progression. Complete cytoreduction may not be possible if tumor nodules are allowed to implant in and along vital structures. It is therefore very important to preoperatively assess the number and extension of prior surgeries before attempting a definitive cytoreductive surgery with perioperative intraperitoneal chemotherapy. PSS has been shown to be an important quantitative prognostic indicator [15]. Patients with no prior abdominopelvic surgery or biopsy only receive a PSS of 0, those with up to one AR dissected receive a PSS of 1, those with two to five AR receive a PSS of 2, and those with six or more regions dissected receive a PSS of 3. The PSS is determined prior to surgical exploration from a review of all prior operative notes. If more than one surgical procedure was performed, the total number of regions dissected at all prior interventions determines the PSS.

The use of the AR shown in Fig. 10.1 not only can define the extent of prior surgery but can be used to quantitate the extent of carcinomatosis.

The PCI is useful for patient selection for a comprehensive treatment plan [16]. The PCI is a quantitative prognostic indicator determined after abdominal exploration and complete separation of intestinal adhesions. This index adds a lesion size parameter within each AR to achieve a numerical score estimating the extent of carcinomatosis. The lesion size score (LS) is used to quantitate the size of peritoneal nodules. LS-0 indicates no tumor visualized, LS-1 indicates tumor implants up to 0.5 cm, LS-2 indicates tumor implants up to 5 cm and LS-3 indicates tumor implants larger than 5 cm or layering of cancer. The summation of the LS in each of the 13 AR is the PCI, ranging from 0 to 39. As discussed later in this chapter, the PCI provides a useful guideline that helps direct the surgeon toward comprehensive treatment when the score is low; a high score would suggest a minimal palliative intervention.

Completeness of cytoreduction (CC) is a quantitative prognostic indicator determined after the surgical resection has been completed. A patient receives a CC-0 score when no visible peritoneal carcinomatosis remains after cytoreduction, CC-1 is recorded when tumor nodules persist after cytoreduction but they measure less than 0.25 cm, CC-2 when remaining tumor measures between 0.25 and 2.5 cm. When tumor nodules are greater than 2.5 cm or there is confluence of unresectable tumor, a CC-3 score is given to the patient. Several prior studies in ovarian cancer have shown that the size of the cancer nodules remaining after cytoreduction is directly related to the survival. The smaller the residual nodules, the greater the likelihood of a long-term survival [17, 18]. By a "log-kill" hypothesis, one would predict this observation to be true. Patients who have a complete cytoreduction have a statistically improved survival when compared to suboptimal cytoreduction [15].

10.5
Surgical Techniques Used to Achieve a Complete Cytoreduction in Selected Patients

The goal of cytoreductive surgery is to reduce the tumor burden within the abdomen and pelvis to its absolute minimal volume. The best result is a patient who is visibly free of disease at the close of the procedure. The surgery combines a series of peritonectomy procedures and visceral resections (Table 10.1). All resections are performed on an as necessary basis; no structures are resected unless they are visibly involved by cancer.

Table 10.1 Visceral resections and peritonectomy procedures that may be required for complete cytoreduction

Cytoreduction	
Visceral resections	**Peritonectomy procedures**
Resection of prior abdominal incisions	Anterior parietal peritonectomy
Greater omentectomy ± splenectomy	Left upper quadrant peritonectomy
Rectosigmoid colon resection	Right upper quadrant peritonectomy
Hysterectomy and oophorectomy	Pelvic peritonectomy
Cholecystectomy	Lesser omentectomy with stripping of the omental bursa

10.5.1
Patient Preparation for Surgery

Once a decision to proceed with surgery is made a surgical conditioning program is initiated. It is advised that the patient adheres to a balanced diet with adequate amount of vitamins and proteins; most important is an exercise regimen that would improve aerobic capabilities and muscular mass.

A routine bowel preparation is prescribed for the day prior to the surgery. Under general endotracheal anesthesia with adequate monitoring (cardiac rhythm, invasive and noninvasive blood pressure, pulse oximetry, central temperature, muscle relaxation), the surgical team introduces a double-lumen central venous line with the purpose of both central venous pressure monitoring and fluids administration. Later in the postoperative period, this line will be used for total parenteral nutrition administration. Both arms are placed in abduction and the back in extension. Sequential compression boots (SBC Compression Boots, Kendall Co., MA) are placed surrounding the calves as prophylaxis against deep venous thrombosis. The surgeon places the lower extremities in the lithotomy position using St. Mark's leg holders (AMSCO, Erie, PA) so that weight of the leg is held by the heels and not by the calves [17]. Soft shoulder braces are used to prevent movement of the patient's body on the operating table when steep Trendelenburg position is used [18]. Because the surgical intervention may last for 8–12 h, it is extremely important to verify that the patient's position on the table is adequate. Postoperative problems caused by decubitus ulcer, temperature extremes, nerve damage, and leg compartment syndromes must be avoided. Egg-crate foam padding for arms and legs and body surface warming devices are used to decrease the risk of such complications.

Antibiotics are administered in a prophylactic fashion. The extension of the raw surfaces after peritonectomies highly increases the risk of postoperative hemorrhage precluding the use of pharmacologic deep vein thrombosis prophylaxis in the first 4 or 5 days postoperatively.

Other requirements for a successful cytoreductive surgery on the operating table are two suction tubes, an electrosurgical unit capable of high voltage pure cut and spray coagulation modes, a 3 mm electrosurgery ball-tip, an electrosurgery tip extender, and at least one smoke evacuator. The temperatures at the electrosurgical dissection plane can be very high. The second assistant or the scrub nurse intermittently irrigates with room temperature normal saline solution in order to cool adjacent tissues and thereby prevent heat necrosis of tubular structures. Also, frequent irrigation keeps tissues clean of debris or blood, thus preserving the transparency of tissues.

Once the surgical field is properly prepared and draped, the Thompson self-retaining retractor's frame is fixed to the operating table (Thompson Surgical Instruments, Inc., Traverse City, MI). The surgeon may fasten suction tubes, electrosurgery cable, and smoke evacuator hoses to the Thompson retractor's frame using plastic bands.

10.6
Anterior Parietal Peritonectomy and Complete Abdominal Exploration

In order to perform a full abdominal exploration a vertical median xipho-pubic incision is performed. The incision should include the umbilicus since, in cases of peritoneal carcinomatosis; this anatomic site is at a very high risk of cancer involvement. When patients want to preserve the umbilicus for esthetic reasons, a plastic reconstruction can be accomplished.

To facilitate the anterior parietal peritonectomy, the incised skin edges are elevated in a symmetrical manner by cutaneous traction on the skin edges [19, 20]. The old abdominal incision is reached and incised (Fig. 10.2). It is dissected away from the underlying anterior parietal peritoneum towards the left and the right of the midline, initially in a centrifugal fashion. Once the dissection has progressed about 5 cm from midline, the self-retaining retractor blades are placed so that they pull back the abdominal wall creating an angle between the peritoneum and the posterior rectus sheath. The initial centripetal dissection continues laterally to the paracolic sulci. In the cephalic direction the resection includes the round and falciform ligaments. In the caudal direction the anterior parietal peritoneum specimen is separated from the pelvic peritoneum at the dome of the bladder.

Once the anterior parietal peritoneum specimen is removed, the surgeon can perform a complete abdominal exploration, which includes lysis of all adhesions. At this time, the PCI can be calculated. The success of complete cytoreduction and long-term survival can be predicted by assessment of the distribution and the mass of peritoneal surface cancer [21]. The PCI is a predictor of the surgeon's ability to achieve an optimal cytoreduction.

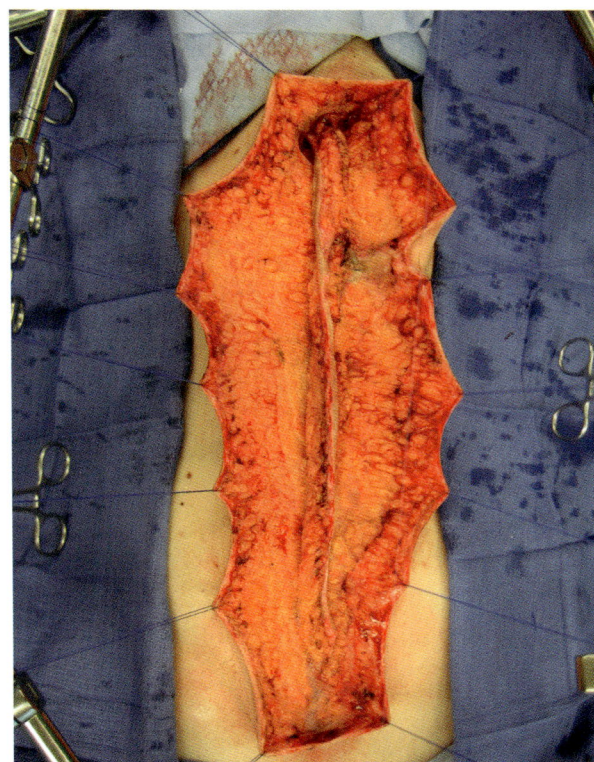

Fig. 10.2 Cutaneous traction sutures are placed using a strong monofilament suture. The sutures are placed approximately every 8 cm along the skin edge. The traction sutures are secured to the self-retaining retractor using hemostats. As the subcutaneous tissue is progressively divided the cutaneous traction sutures are pulled higher onto the self-retaining retractor. With permission from Sugarbaker [19]

10.7
Right and Left Subphrenic Peritonectomies

The right subphrenic peritonectomy is part of a centripetal dissection that starts by detaching the peritoneum from the undersurface of the right hemidiaphragm [22]. It is also necessary to detach the peritoneum from the liver surface and to electroevaporate any disease from Glisson's capsule. Behind the liver, the dissection extends centripetally to the inferior vena cava. The peritoneum covering the perirenal fat and the right adrenal gland is also detached from the posteroinferior edge of the liver. The duodenum and the porta hepatis constitute the medial border of the right subphrenic peritonectomy (Fig. 10.3).

In a similar centripetal fashion, the left subphrenic peritonectomy includes the undersurface of the left hemidiaphragm, dissection of the left lobe of the liver from the triangular ligament which becomes a part of the peritonectomy specimen, and electroevaporation of the left lobe Glisson's capsule. This dissection liberates the spleen which at this point in time remains attached to its pedicle, to the greater omentum and to the lienocolic ligament.

The surgeon must avoid penetrating the diaphragm if at all possible. Diaphragm perforation will allow cancer dissemination into the thoracic cavity. In case of diaphragm penetration, the defect should be enlarged to excise all diaphragm involved by cancer. The HIPEC should be allowed to enter the chest cavity through a generous diaphragmatic incision in an attempt to prevent pleural implantation. The closure of the diaphragm should take place after the HIPEC plus is finished.

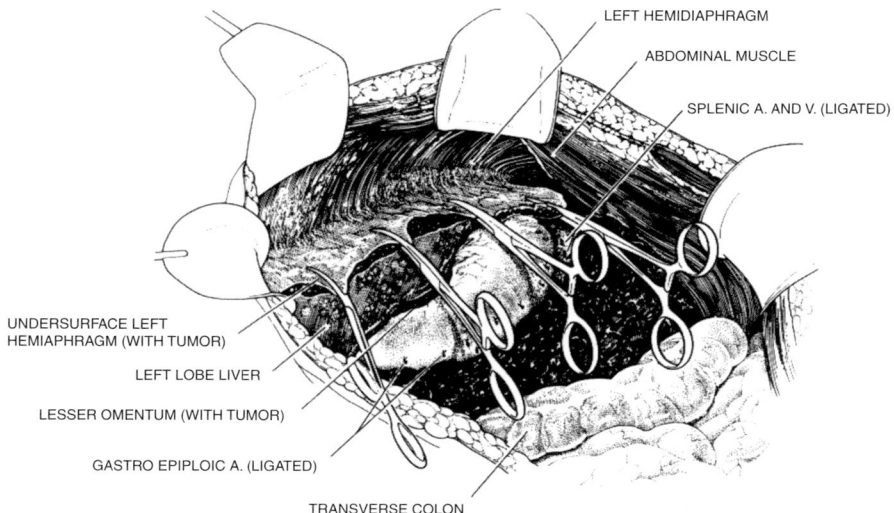

LEFT HEMIDIAPHRAGM

ABDOMINAL MUSCLE

SPLENIC A. AND V. (LIGATED)

UNDERSURFACE LEFT
HEMIAPHRAGM (WITH TUMOR)

LEFT LOBE LIVER

LESSER OMENTUM (WITH TUMOR)

GASTRO EPIPLOIC A. (LIGATED)

TRANSVERSE COLON

Fig. 10.3 Right subphrenic peritonectomy. With permission from Sugarbaker [22]

10.8
Greater and Lesser Omentectomy

The greater omentum is detached from the transverse colon along with the visceral perito-neum that covers the anterior aspect of the transverse colon mesentery. The right gastro-epiploic artery is ligated in continuity and all the small gastroepiploic branches on the greater curvature are also individually ligated as they reach the stomach. The short gastric vessels are also dissected and sectioned. At this point it is necessary to carefully evaluate the splenic hilum, which is a prominent site for cancer deposits. If the spleen or its hilum appears to be involved, splenic artery and veins are individualized and ligated. In order to complete the greater omentectomy, the left gastroepiploic vessel is ligated in continuity and divided.

The pancreas needs to be protected from trauma, especially when dissecting the splenic vessels.

10.9
Pelvic Peritonectomy with Rectosigmoid Colon Resection

The stripping of the pelvic peritoneum always includes the peritoneum of the cul-de-sac (Fig. 10.4). Before starting the dissection the surgeon must evaluate the status of the sig-moid colon and rectum. The epiploic appendages contain a large amount of lymphoid aggregates which have great absorptive capabilities similar to those of the greater omen-tum, making it possible that these appendages will have a large volume of tumor. This and the fact that the peritoneal cul-de-sac is intimately attached to the rectum, frequently make it impossible for the surgeon to make the patient disease-free without a rectosigmoid resection along with the pelvic peritonectomy.

The centripetal dissection for the pelvic peritonectomy starts by separating it from the bladder with the creation of an anterior flap of peritoneum. The posterior flap of perito-neum starts at the area of the ligament of Treitz. There, the posterior parietal peritoneum is separated from the fourth portion of duodenum; the inferior mesenteric vein is ligated in continuity, and the dissection progresses medially separating the peritoneum from the third portion of the duodenum. The stripping proceeds caudally as the colon is divided at the junction of descending and sigmoid regions with a linear stapler, and the inferior mesen-teric artery is ligated and sectioned. On the right side of the abdomen, the terminal ileum and the right colon are freed, and the posterior parietal peritoneum is divided from the colon and ileum. Both ovarian veins are ligated and divided at the level of the inferior border of the perirenal fat. Left and right ureters have to be identified as peritoneal strip-ping continues towards the pelvis. Laterally, the uterine arteries are ligated superior to the ureters and the dissection meets the lateral aspect of the rectum below the peritoneal cul-de-sac. The anterior pelvic peritonectomy proceeds to the vagina which is divided from the uterus and cervix reaching the anterior aspect of the rectum. Once the circumferential electroevaporation has freed up the rectum, the organ is divided with a linear stapler at the

Fig. 10.4 Complete pelvic
peritonectomy. With
permission from
Sugarbaker [22]

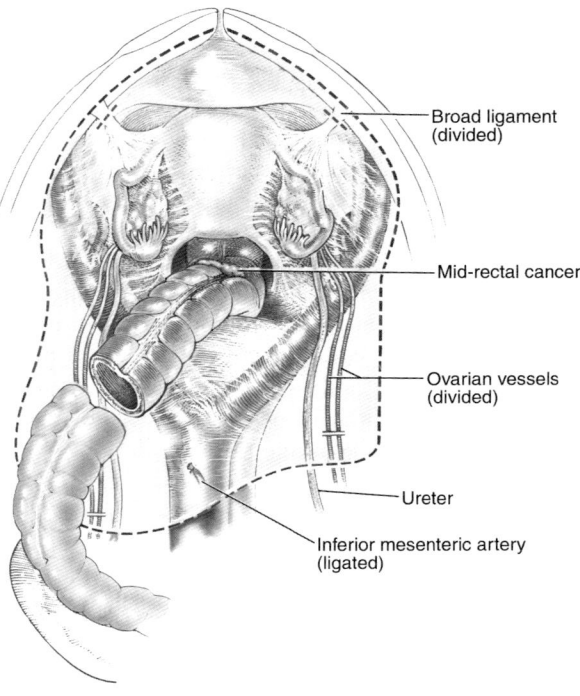

Broad ligament
(divided)

Mid-rectal cancer

Ovarian vessels
(divided)

Ureter

Inferior mesenteric artery
(ligated)

junction of the middle and upper third of the rectum. The specimen of pelvic peritonectomy contains the pelvic peritoneum, the rectosigmoid colon and the upper portion of the
rectum, and if not previously extirpated the uterus and ovaries.

10.10
Rationale for Heated Intraoperative Intraperitoneal Chemotherapy and Early Postoperative Intraperitoneal Chemotherapy

After the abdomen and pelvis have been made visibly free of disease, an immense number
of cancer cells invisible to the naked eye, remain within the peritoneal cavity. Tumor
manipulation, transected lymphatic ducts and small veins leaking tumor cells throughout
the procedure, and small tumor nodules remaining on the abdominal and pelvic surfaces of
organs not amenable to peritonectomy procedures, namely small bowel, require the implementation of some method that will eradicate residual tumor cells. Another well known
site for persistent disease is the suture lines that are an ideal site for cancer cell implants.
Tumor cell entrapment occurs on these raw surfaces with fibrin accumulating and tissues
compressed together by stitches or staples. Suture lines are at high risk for recurrence if
constructed before the HIPEC plus.

HIPEC plus, using an open technique, employs mechanical, physical and chemical effects to eradicate residual cancer cells after cytoreductive surgery. A mechanical effect to eradicate cancer cells trapped in fibrin and tissue debris takes place during 90 min of continuous rubbing and washing of the intraabdominal surfaces. Heat, a physical effect, promotes cell death by various mechanisms affecting nucleic acids, cell membranes and the cytoskeleton [23]. The target temperature within the peritoneal cavity is approximately 42°C. Some chemotherapeutic agents such as mitomycin C, doxorubicin, cisplatin, and melphalan among others, have their cell killing effect enhanced by heat [24]. Also, penetration of chemotherapy into tissues is augmented by heat [25].

The intraperitoneal route of chemotherapy administration has another advantage. The concentration times time (area under the curve or AUC) of the cytotoxic agent in the peritoneal cavity is many times higher than that in the plasma compartment. The AUC ratio of peritoneal to plasma varies for different drugs; for example, it can be as high as 1,000 for paclitaxel [26]. This feature of intraperitoneal chemotherapy with selected drugs makes possible high concentration of the agent where the disease is localized, enhancing the cell killing effect and decreasing the systemic toxicity. Ideally, the drug to be used should be active against ovarian cancer, nontoxic for noncancer cells, of high molecular weight to allow a low peritoneal clearance, and have a high penetration into tumor tissues.

Several drugs have been used for intraperitoneal irrigation for patients with ovarian cancer: cisplatin alone, carboplatin alone, mitoxantrone alone and cisplatin plus doxorubicin [27–30]. Our group has used a combination of cisplatin (50 mg/m^2) and doxorubicin (15 mg/m^2). Sugarbaker, after a dose escalation study, determined that a low dose of doxorubicin (15 mg/m^2) would result in a thin layering of fibrous tissue on peritoneal surfaces that has not been reported to interfere in any way with subsequent gastrointestinal function [31].

There are multiple reasons to recommend doxorubicin as an intraperitoneal chemotherapy agent [32]. Perhaps most important, due to the large molecular size of this drug its clearance from the peritoneal cavity is greatly delayed. It is also known that its penetration is at least five cell layers making it appropriate for the elimination of small volume residual disease postoperatively. It is also augmented in its anticancer effects by heat [25]. A unique characteristic of hyperthermic intraperitoneal doxorubicin is its accumulation within cancerous tissue at concentrations greater than the concentration of the chemotherapy solution. Apparently, doxorubicin binds irreversibly to intracellular proteins [33].

Cisplatin has been shown to have improved penetration into cancerous tissue when administered with heat as compared to normothermic conditions. The increase in cytotoxicity is estimated at 1.8 times [34]. Also, the peritoneum/plasma AUC ratio is favorable; however, hypothermia does increase the renal toxicity potential of cisplatin. These factors plus the activity of this drug, both for primary and recurrent ovarian cancer has led to its frequent use in intraperitoneal administration [35].

Simultaneously, with the administration of intraperitoneal cisplatin and doxorubicin, ifosfamide is given intravenously. This is a drug with a large amount of increased cytotoxicity with heat [36]. The theoretical basis for intravenous ifosfamide to be used for peritoneal carcinomatosis is heat targeting. The tissues immediately adjacent to the peritoneal space are heated; the ifosfamide in these tissues will, therefore, have enhanced toxicity. These are the surfaces that contain minute cancerous deposits that need to be eradicated.

10.10.1
Technique for Heated Intraoperative Intraperitoneal Chemotherapy

An abdominopelvic reservoir is constructed by tenting up the skin edges to a specially designed instrument that allows hand distribution of the chemotherapy agent and total containment [37] (Fig. 10.5). The double-gloved hand guarantees that the perfusate reaches all surfaces within the peritoneal cavity, such as the space between the bowel loops, the space behind the liver, and the pelvic cavity.

In order to keep the temperature at a constant 42°C, a roller pump forces the solution through a heat exchanger. Then it proceeds into the abdominopelvic cavity through a Tenckhoff catheter. The hyperthermic perfusate is drained from the abdomen through four closed drains going back to the heat exchanger, and closing the circuit. The Tenckhoff catheter and the closed suction drains are secured watertight with purse-string sutures on the skin of the abdomen to avoid leaks and spillage. The chemotherapy solution circulates for 90 min at 42°C.

After the 90 min of HIPEC plus with manual distribution, the surgeon may assume that fibrin, tissue debris, and the microscopic residual disease they contain have been eradicated. At this time, all the anastomoses and any additional reconstruction can occur. The

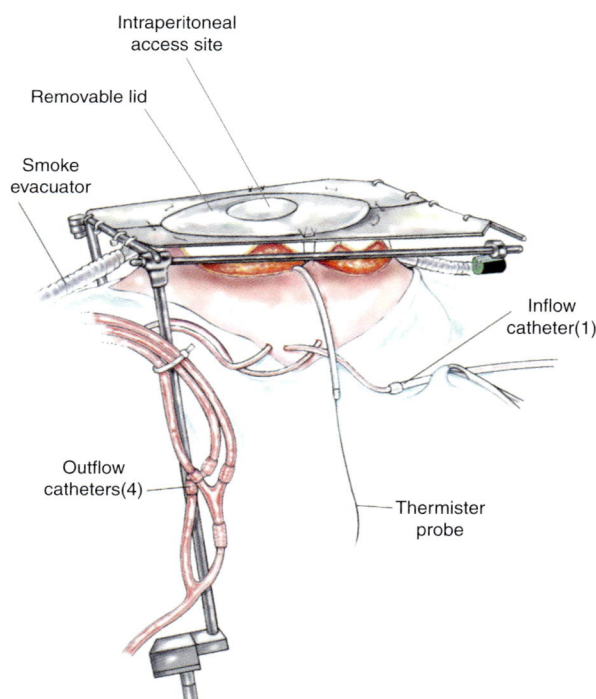

Fig. 10.5 Intraoperative administration of intraperitoneal chemotherapy. With permission from Sugarbaker [37]

same closed-suction drains and inflow catheters used for HIPEC plus are properly positioned for subsequent EPIC with paclitaxel.

10.10.2
Technique for Early Perioperative Intraperitoneal Chemotherapy

In the first 5 postoperative days the patient receives normothermic intraperitoneal paclitaxel (20–40 mg/m^2/day), with the goal of consolidating the intraperitoneal chemotherapy treatments. Systemic paclitaxel has been used to treat advanced ovarian cancer alone and in combination with other drugs. In phase III clinical trials the combination resulted in improved response rates and also improved survival [11]. The extremely favorable AUC ratio and the remarkable drug penetration of up to 80 cell layers deserve mention [38].

Mohamed and colleagues studied the use of paclitaxel in 6% hetastarch as a carrier solution [39]. The retention of the high molecular weight carrier solution as compared to the salt solution in the abdominopelvic space improved the drug exposure to peritoneal surface cancer nodules without any increase in systemic toxicity.

A potential problem with intraperitoneal paclitaxel is the lipid solvent and the fact that carcinogens can be leached out of soft plastic used to administer the infusions. Stuart and colleagues discussed the technical precautions that will minimize this potential hazard [40].

In summary, HIPEC plus and EPIC combine mechanical, physical and chemical effects to eradicate microscopic residual disease. They are used as a planned part of the surgical procedure and the postoperative care in the highly controlled environments of the operating room, surgical intensive care unit, and a specialized nursing unit.

10.10.3
Modifications of Surgical Practice with Cytoreduction and Multiagent Perioperative Chemotherapy

In the program of management currently active at the Washington Cancer Institute, four chemotherapy agents discussed previously (cisplatin, doxorubicin, ifosfamide and paclitaxel), all with high response rates for ovarian cancer, are used as a planned essential part of comprehensive management.

This multiagent chemotherapy along with the cytoreductive surgery demands some modifications of the surgical procedure. Undoubtedly, in the comprehensive management plan the generous use of a diverting ostomy is necessary. Anastomotic disruption with fistula can occur as a result of the delayed wound healing expected in these patients. In patients who have a low colorectal anastomosis but no other bowel resections, our current practice is to plicate the bowel around the stapled anastomosis to form a two-layer colorectal closure. If the anastomosis is too low in the rectum to allow such a second layer, then a diverting ileostomy should be performed. If there are more than two anastomoses required, the most proximal segment of bowel should be exteriorized as a temporary ileostomy.

10.11
Results of Comprehensive Treatment in Advanced
Primary and Recurrent Ovarian Cancer

In patients who have failed the standard treatments for primary ovarian cancer survival is short with an estimated median survival of 9 months. Figure 10.6 presents the survival of 28 patients with greatly advanced primary (4 patients) and recurrent epithelial ovarian cancer (24 patients) who had an attempt at complete cytoreduction at the Washington Cancer Institute. Median survival was 45.8 months [15]. Further analysis by Look and colleagues showed that extent of prior surgery and completeness of cytoreduction were independent factors significantly affecting survival [15]. Patients with extensive prior surgery (e.g., with three or more AR subjected to surgical dissection) were less likely to receive a complete cytoreduction and their survival was significantly shorter. Patients with a low PSS who had less than three AR previously dissected had a median survival of 6.5 years, compared to 1.5 years for those patients with a higher PSS ($p < 0.001$). Patients with an adequate cytoreduction had a median survival of 55.9 months; suboptimal cytoreduction showed an 8 month survival ($p = 0.037$).

At this point in time, a precise response rate to the hyperthermic bidirectional multiagent perioperative chemotherapy regimen is not available. However, anecdotal assessments of response using histologic criteria in patients having a second look surgery are available. Figure 10.7 shows a histologic section of a high grade papillary serous adenocarcinoma; psammomatous calcifications are present. At a second look surgery approximately 1 year later with no additional treatment, the epithelial component of the cancer has disappeared. Only the psammomatous calcifications remain within a background of fibrous tissue (Fig. 10.8).

Tentes and colleagues reported on the PCI as a quantitative prognostic indicator in 60 women with ovarian cancer [16]. Those patients with a PCI lower than 10 had a median

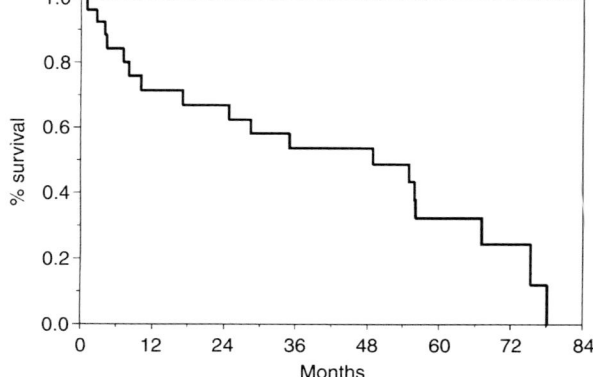

Fig. 10.6 Overall survival of 28 patients given comprehensive treatment for recurrent ovarian cancer. With permission from Look et al. [15]

Fig. 10.7 Photomicrograph of a papillary serous adenocarcinoma with psammomatous calcifications in a 54 year old woman. The patient was treated with cytoreductive surgery plus hyperthermic bidirectional perioperative chemotherapy (Hematoxylin and eosin ×40)

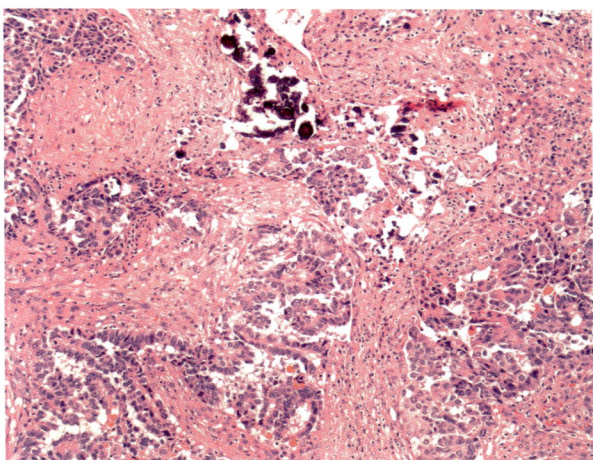

Fig. 10.8 Photomicrograph of a papillary serous adenocarcinoma approximately 1 year later at second-look surgery. The epithelial component of the disease has been eradicated and the psammomatous calcifications remain in a background of fibrous tissue

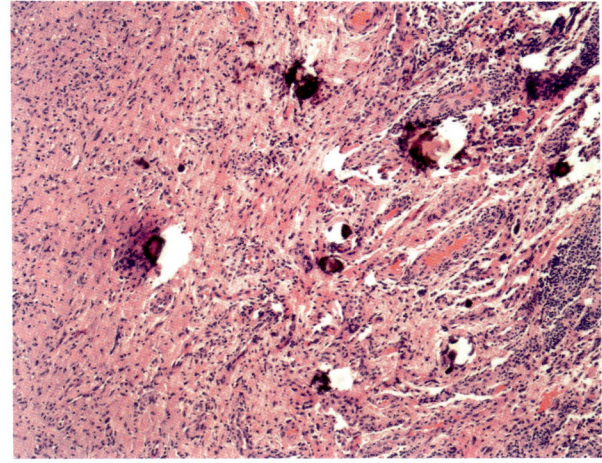

survival of 80 months and a 5-year survival of 65%, while those patients with a PCI greater than 10 had a median survival of 38 months and a 5-year survival rate of 29% ($p=0.0253$).

Recently, Bijelic and colleagues published a systematic review analyzing 14 studies that reported on cytoreduction and hyperthermic intraperitoneal chemotherapy. Ten studies reported a positive impact on survival and survival was not analyzed in four studies. Morbidity ranged from 5 to 36% and the median mortality was 3% [41].

10.12
Morbidity and Mortality

The combination of cytoreductive surgery and perioperative intraperitoneal chemotherapy, as previously described is associated with 20% of patients experiencing morbidity and with a 2% mortality rate [42]. The typical postoperative course for patients at Washington University involves an average 21-day hospital stay. They usually have a prolonged ileus lasting for 10–14 days. Nasogastric suction is sustained until the bowel function is recovered. All patients receive total parenteral nutrition while intestinal function is negligible. After the nasogastric tube is withdrawn oral nutrition is gradually resumed over approximately 1 week. The most common complications are central line infections (12%), pancreatitis (4%) and intestinal fistulas (3%). Anastomotic leak rate is 2%.

10.13
The Peritoneum as a First Line of Defense Against Carcinomatosis

Our current hypothesis regarding proper treatment of ovarian cancer considers the peritoneum as the human body's first line of defense against carcinomatosis. Whenever the peritoneum is violated by surgery, residual cancer cells are implanted and then progress beyond the peritoneum. In the abdomen or pelvis with a high PSS the peritonectomy becomes technically much more difficult or impossible. Also, tumor growth deep into the peritoneum at crucial anatomic sites increases the likelihood of severe complications, such as ureteral and vascular injuries during surgery and intestinal fistulas presenting in the postoperative period. The pelvic side wall after pelvic lymph node dissection presents a special problem.

In any surgery for ovarian cancer involving stripping of peritoneal surfaces, there is a high likelihood of malignant seeding. My opinion is that an attempt should be made at eradicating all tumors to prevent further cancer cell contamination and microscopic residual disease [15]. This approach employs proper "respect for the peritoneum" in patients with carcinomatosis. Complete tumor removal and then perioperative chemotherapy are essential parts of the strategy used to achieve this goal.

10.14
Comparison of Ovarian and Appendiceal Cancer

A similar clinical situation to ovarian cancer is appendiceal cancer. With an unruptured primary tumor, the prognosis of both ovarian cancer and a malignant mucocoele is excellent with near 100% survival with simple excision. However, if peritoneal seeding has occurred the prognosis changes dramatically and a curative treatment plan requires cytoreductive surgery and perioperative intraperitoneal chemotherapy. A difference in appendiceal mucinous neoplasms as compared to ovarian cancer is a remarkably low incidence of lymph node metastases (4%) as compared to near 50% for stage III ovarian cancer [43]. The results of treatment are, therefore, more favorable with appendiceal cancer. These advanced appendiceal cancer results have been summarized in a collective review by Yan et al. [44]. Ten recent manuscripts from experienced groups reported 5-year survival of 52–96%. The morbidity varied from 33 to 56% and mortality 0 to 18% [44]. Sugarbaker compared comprehensive treatment of pseudomyxoma peritonei to serial debulking with or without systemic chemotherapy [45]. The comprehensive management showed 75% survival at 20 years; three other prominent institutions had near 0% survival at 20 years. High grade appendiceal cancer has shown a 40% survival at 5 years [46].

10.15
Conclusions

This highly specialized treatment needs to be performed by qualified surgeons who are knowledgeable about intraperitoneal chemotherapy administration as well as the complications of this comprehensive management plan. Accepting the fact that there might be a selection bias, the results with this comprehensive treatment are encouraging. A multiinstitutional phase II study is indicated to validate these results in patients with recurrent ovarian cancer. Its role in treatment of primary disease will be its best application.

References

1. Surveillance, Epidemiology, and End Results (SEER) Program (2001) SEER* Stat database: SEER incidence – AA rates for White/Black/Other, 1973-2001. National Cancer Institute, DCCPS, Surveillance Research Program, Cancer Statistics Branch, Bethesda, MD
2. Surveillance, Epidemiology, and End Results (SEER) Program (2001) SEER* Stat database: US estimated complete prevalence counts on 1/1/2001. National Cancer Institute, DCCPS, Surveillance Research Program, Cancer Statistics Branch, Bethesda, MD
3. Surveillance, Epidemiology, and End Results (SEER) Program (2003) SEER* Stat database: 12 registries incidence and mortality. National Cancer Institute, DCCPS, Surveillance Research Program, Cancer Statistics Branch, Bethesda, MD
4. Parkin DM, Pisani P, Ferlay J (1999) Estimates of the worldwide incidence of 25 major cancers in 1990. Int J Cancer 80:827–841
5. Goff BA, Mandel LS, Melancon CH, Muntz HG (2004) Frequency of symptoms of ovarian cancer in women presenting to primary care clinics. JAMA 291:2705–2712
6. Schapira MM, Matchar DB, Young MJ (1993) The effectiveness of ovarian cancer screening. A decision analysis model. Ann Intern Med 118:838–843
7. Sampson J (1931) Implantation peritoneal carcinomatosis of ovarian origin. J Pathol VII:423–443
8. Carmignani CP, Sugarbaker TA, Bromley CM, Sugarbaker PH (2003) Intraperitoneal cancer dissemination: mechanisms of the patterns of spread. Cancer Metastasis Rev 22:465–472
9. Delgado G, Chun B, Caglar H, Bepko F (1977) Paraaortic lymphadenectomy in gynecologic malignancies confined to the pelvis. Obstet Gynecol 50:418–423

10. Alberts DS, Liu PY, Hannigan EV et al (1996) Intraperitoneal cisplatin plus intravenous cyclophosphamide versus intravenous cisplatin plus intravenous cyclophosphamide for stage III ovarian cancer. N Engl J Med 335:1950–1955

11. Markman M, Bundy BN, Alberts DS et al (2001) Phase III trial of standard-dose intravenous cisplatin plus paclitaxel versus moderately high-dose carboplatin followed by intravenous paclitaxel and intraperitoneal cisplatin in small-volume stage III ovarian carcinoma: an intergroup study of the Gynecologic Oncology Group, Southwestern Oncology Group, and Eastern Cooperative Oncology Group. J Clin Oncol 19:1001–1007

12. Armstrong DK, Bundy B, Wenzel L et al (2006) Intraperitoneal cisplatin and paclitaxel in ovarian cancer. N Engl J Med 354:34–43

13. Gonzalez Bayon L, Sugarbaker PH, Gonzalez Moreno S et al (2003) Initiation of a program in peritoneal surface malignancy. Surg Oncol Clin N Am 12:741–753

14. Jacquet P, Sugarbaker PH (1996) Current methodologies for clinical assessment of patients with peritoneal carcinomatosis. J Exp Clin Cancer Res 15:49–58

15. Look M, Chang D, Sugarbaker PH (2003) Long-term results of cytoreductive surgery for advanced and recurrent epithelial ovarian cancers and papillary serous carcinoma of the peritoneum. Int J Gynecol Cancer 13:764–770

16. Tentes AAK, Tripsiannis G, Markakidis SK et al (2003) Peritoneal cancer index: a prognostic indicator of survival in advanced ovarian cancer. Eur J Surg Oncol 29:69–73

17. Young R, Perez C, Hoskins W (1993) Cancer of the ovary. In: DeVita V, Hellman S (eds) Cancer: principles and practice of oncology. JB Lippincott, Philadelphia, PA, p 1226

18. Zang RY, Zhang ZY, Li ZT et al (2000) Impact of secondary cytoreductive surgery on survival of patients with advanced epithelial ovarian cancer. Eur J Surg Oncol 26:798–804

19. Sugarbaker PH (2008) Circumferential cutaneous traction for exposure of the layers of the abdominal wall. J Surg Oncol 98:472–475

20. De Lima Vazquez V, Sugarbaker PH (2003) Total anterior parietal peritonectomy. J Surg Oncol 83:261–263

21. Esquivel J, Farinetti A, Sugarbaker PH (1999) Elective surgery in recurrent colon cancer with peritoneal seeding: when to and when not to proceed. G Chir 20:81–86

22. Sugarbaker PH (1995) Peritonectomy procedures. Ann Surg 221:29–42

23. Christophi C, Winkworth A, Muralihdaran V, Evans P (1998) The treatment of malignancy by hyperthermia. Surg Oncol 7:83–90

24. Takahashi I, Emi Y, Hasuda S et al (2002) Clinical application of hyperthermia combined with anticancer drugs for the treatment of solid tumors. Surgery 131:S78–S84

25. Jacquet P, Averbach A, Stuart OA et al (1998) Hyperthermic intraperitoneal doxorubicin: pharmacokinetics, metabolism, and tissue distribution in a rat model. Cancer Chemother Pharmacol 41:147–154

26. Markman M, Rowinsky E, Hakes T et al (1992) Phase I trial of intraperitoneal taxol: a Gynecoloic Oncology Group study. J Clin Oncol 10:1485–1491

27. van der Vange N, van Goethem AR, Zoetmulder FA et al (2000) Extensive cytoreductive surgery combined with intra-operative intraperitoneal perfusion with cisplatin under hyperthermic conditions (OVHIPEC) in patients with recurrent ovarian cancer: a feasibility pilot. Eur J Surg Oncol 26:663–668

28. Steller MA, Egorin MJ, Trimble EL et al (1999) A pilot phase I trial of continuous hyperthermic peritoneal perfusion with high-dose carboplatin as primary treatment of patients with small-volume residual ovarian cancer. Cancer Chemother Pharmacol 43:106–114

29. Nicoletto MO, Padrini R, Galeotti F et al (2000) Pharmacokinetics of intraperitoneal hyperthermic perfusion with mitoxantrone in ovarian cancer. Cancer Chemother Pharmacol 45:457–462

30. Deraco M, Rossi CR, Pennacchioli E et al (2001) Cytoreductive surgery followed by intraperitoneal hyperthermic perfusion in the treatment of recurrent epithelial ovarian cancer: a phase II clinical study. Tumori 87:120–126

31. Sugarbaker PH (1996) Early postoperative intraperitoneal adriamycin as an adjuvant treatment for visceral and retroperitoneal sarcoma. In: Sugarbaker PH (ed) Peritoneal carcinomatosis: drugs and diseases. Kluwer, Boston, MA, pp 15–30

32. Ozols RF, Locker GY, Doroshow JH et al (1979) Pharmacokinetics of adriamycin and tissue penetration in murine ovarian cancer. Cancer Res 39:3209–3214

33. Van der Speeten K, Stuart OA, Mahteme H, Sugarbaker PH (2009) A pharmacologic analysis of intraoperative intracavitary cancer chemotherapy with doxorubicin. Cancer Chemother Pharmacol 63:799–805

34. Los G, Sminia P, Wondergem J et al (1991) Optimisation of intraperitoneal cisplatin therapy with regional hyperthermia in rats. Eur J Cancer 27:472–477

35. Panteix G, Beaujard A, Garbit F et al (2002) Population pharmacokinetics of cisplatin in patients with advanced ovarian cancer during intraperitoneal hyperthermia chemotherapy. Anticancer Res 22:1329–1336

36. Urano M, Kuroda M, Nishimura Y (1999) Invited review for the clinical application of thermochemotherapy given at mild temperatures. Int J Hyperthermia 15:79–107

37. Sugarbaker PH (2005) An instrument to provide containment of intraoperative intraperitoneal chemotherapy with optimized distribution. J Surg Oncol 92:142–146

38. Kuh H, Jang SH, Wientjes MG et al (1999) Determinants of paclitaxel penetration and accumulation in human solid tumor. J Pharmacol Exp Ther 290:871–880

39. Mohamed F, Marchettini P, Stuart OA, Sugarbaker PH (2003) Pharmacokinetics and tissue distribution of intraperitoneal paclitaxel with different carrier solutions. Cancer Chemother Pharmacol 52:405–410

40. Stuart OA, Knight C, Sugarbaker PH (2005) Avoiding carcinogen exposure with intraperitoneal paclitaxel. Oncol Nurs Forum 32:44–48

41. Bijelic L, Jonson A, Sugarbaker PH (2007) Systematic review of cytoreductive surgery and heated intraoperative intraperitoneal chemotherapy for treatment of peritoneal carcinomatosis in primary and recurrent ovarian cancer. Ann Oncol 18:1943–1950

42. Yan TD, Zappa L, Edwards G, Alderman R, Marquardt CE, Sugarbaker PH (2007) Perioperative outcomes of cytoreductive surgery and perioperative intraperitoneal chemotherapy for non-appendiceal peritoneal carcinomatosis from a prospective database. J Surg Oncol 96:102–112

43. Gonzalez-Moreno S, Sugarbaker PH (2004) Right hemicolectomy does not confer a survival advantage in patients with mucinous carcinoma of the appendix and peritoneal seeding. Br J Surg 91:304–311

44. Yan TD, Black D, Savady R, Sugarbaker PH (2007) A systematic review on the efficacy of cytoreductive surgery and perioperative intraperitoneal chemotherapy for pseudomyxoma peritonei. Ann Surg Oncol 14:484–492

45. Sugarbaker PH (2006) New standard of care for appendiceal epithelial neoplasms and pseudomyxoma peritonei syndrome? Lancet Oncol 7:69–76

46. Sugarbaker PH, Chang D (1999) Results of treatment of 385 patients with peritoneal surface spread of appendiceal malignancy. Ann Surg Oncol 6:727–731

Health-Related Quality of Life and Patient-Reported Outcomes

11

Lisa M. Hess

11.1
Introduction

The World Health Organization (WHO) in its constitution defines health as "a state of complete physical, mental and social well-being and not merely the absence of disease or infirmity" [1]. Increasingly, health is no longer being measured exclusively by the clinical features of disease. Family, caregiver, and patient-reported health outcomes are gaining importance from the earliest phases of clinical research to the implementation of public health policies. Health outcomes are no longer limited to survival or mortality, but now include many aspects of well-being, such as morbidity, comfort, satisfaction, psychosocial function, social support, health status, clinical factors, and economic factors [2].

As health care transitions from a directive approach to a more patient-centered model of care, clinicians and researchers now view direct inquiry of the patient's perspective of their own well-being to be the best source of information about how the patient is feeling, rather than relying exclusively on patient observation. Patients are a key source of information about how they are feeling during and following treatment. The direct elicitation of information from the patient falls into the broad category of patient-reported outcomes (PROs), which refers to any outcome that is assessed from the patient's perspective. PROs are of particular concern in the care of women who have been diagnosed with ovarian cancer. Unlike many other cancers, there is no screening test for ovarian cancer, and it tends to be diagnosed at advanced stages (more than 75% of cases are stage III–IV at initial diagnosis) [3]. This contributes to the increased morbidity and mortality associated with diagnosis and a high likelihood of disease recurrence following successful treatment. The majority of women diagnosed with ovarian cancer will live with this cancer for the rest of their lives.

Cancer diagnosis and treatment are very physically challenging, and patients may experience physical, psychological, and social sequelae related to both the disease and its treatment (e.g., acute and chronic cardiac, neurological, and other bodily impairments, economic challenges, emotional concerns, and family issues) [4]. Many cancer patients

L.M. Hess
Indiana University School of Medicine,
714 N Senate Ave., Indianapolis, IN 46202 USA
e-mail: lmhess@iupui.edu

D.S. Alberts et al. (eds.), *Intraperitoneal Therapy for Ovarian Cancer*,
DOI: 10.1007/978-3-642-12130-2_11, © Springer-Verlag Berlin Heidelberg 2010

experience significant physical limitations in their daily living during treatment; however, cancer survivors also may experience persistent functional disabilities following treatment. These challenges can impact an individual's ability to work and to participate in daily, as well as social (e.g., family and community), activities. Women who have been diagnosed with ovarian cancer have reported ongoing psychosocial concerns including fear, coping, and distress, specifically related to family and relationship roles, and the need for social support, in addition to the physical and mortality concerns associated with this cancer and its treatment [5, 6]. Some of the symptoms that may be of particular concern to women treated for ovarian cancer include gastrointestinal toxicities, including abdominal pain, nausea and vomiting, neurotoxicity, hair loss, and fatigue [5, 7–9]. Many of these concerns are best assessed by asking the patient directly, rather than relying on external assessments or clinical measurements. The effects of pain and fear, for example, emphasize the need to include PROs in patient evaluations, whether in research or routine practice. Pain (biologic outcome of cancer) and fear (psychosocial outcome of cancer) are both practically impossible to evaluate without the patient's perspective.

Cancer has a very broad impact that reaches far beyond the person receiving the diagnosis. Family and friends may provide cancer patients with both emotional (e.g., empathy) and practical support (e.g., transportation) during and following treatment, requiring resources (time, energy, money) that would have been used for the family/community to instead support the patient. When a person is diagnosed with cancer, others often assume responsibility for tasks previously performed by the patient [10]. Family income and community productivity may be impacted due to the loss of the ability to work [11]. Family members who were previously cared for may become the caregivers themselves, thus their own quality of life (QOL) is directly impacted by the experience of the family member or friend who received the cancer diagnosis [12, 13]. Husbands and partners of women with ovarian cancer, in particular, experience a variety of emotional, psychological, and social effects due to their own experience with their loved one's cancer [14]. A cancer diagnosis, therefore, affects more than just the patient. By reducing the burden of the disease on the patient, it is possible to improve the well-being of not only the patient, but of her community (friends and family). Due to the increasing cancer incidence and mortality in a setting with increasingly limited resources, it is important to reduce the burden of this disease to the fullest extent possible.

As ovarian cancer care extends beyond the immediate treatment of the disease to include the broader physical and psychosocial aspects of a patient's well-being, research and assessment of PROs are becoming more and more critical to providing women with quality care. As described earlier, patient-reported heath outcomes are any outcome of care that is assessed from the patient's perspective. In general, *health outcomes* are defined as "a change in a patient's current and future health status that can be attributed to antecedent health care" [15]. Health outcomes assessment measures how health care or health interventions may impact a patient's life in a more comprehensive manner than is possible by clinical response assessment alone. Health outcomes fall into three general categories: clinical, economic, and humanistic [16]. Clinical outcomes of care include survival, toxicity, tumor response, biomedical markers such as CA-125 levels, and other factors that can be assessed clinically. Economic outcomes of care include costs of care to the patient, providers, payers, and society. Economic outcomes can include the direct medical costs of care (e.g., physician time, pharmaceuticals, hospital costs), the indirect costs of care (e.g., caregiver time, lost wages, premature mortality), as well as intangible costs (such as pain, suffering, and quality of life). Humanistic outcomes refer to those outcomes as experienced and perceived by the patient.

QOL is one category of humanistic, patient-reported health outcomes. QOL has traditionally been defined very broadly, as one's general perception or overall sense of well-being [17]. Unlike health outcomes, which include both objective (clinically/socially measurable or observable) and subjective (patient-reported) outcomes, QOL cannot be measured by any clinical criteria. QOL is a subjective interpretation of either general (inclusive of all domains) or specific domains of well-being. The domains of QOL include physical, social, psychological, and spiritual well-being [5]. Examples of factors within the domains of QOL and of health outcomes are compared in Table 11.1. Each of these factors may or may not be a PRO, depending on how the information is collected. It is important to note that both for health outcomes and QOL, there are factors external to the individual (e.g., culture, social determinants of health, environment, education, demographics) that must be taken into consideration as well [2].

Table 11.1 Comparison of health outcomes and quality of life [5, 16]

Health outcomes		Quality of life	
Clinical	Results of laboratory tests (e.g., CA-125, hemoglobin) Results of other clinical tests (e.g., CT scan) Toxicities Disease response/progression Survival	**Physical well-being**	Strength/fatigue Sleep/rest Physical health Pain Appetite Other symptoms of treatment (e.g., neuropathy, gastrointestinal)
Humanistic	Quality of life Preferences/values Satisfaction Service utilization Decision-making Patient and caregiver needs	**Social well-being**	Family Roles/relationships Sexuality/fertility Isolation Finances Work Social support
Economic	Direct medical costs (medical resource costs) Direct nonmedical costs (e.g., transportation, housing) Indirect costs (household costs, caregiver time, lost productivity costs) Intangibles (pain and suffering)	**Psychological well-being**	FearControl Anxiety/depression Happiness Cognition Distress Coping Usefulness
		Spiritual well-being	Meaning of illness Religion Spirituality Hope Uncertainty Purpose Outlook

QOL is often more specifically termed health-related quality of life (HRQOL) when it is used to specify the aspects of QOL that are impacted by a health condition or its treatment. HRQOL focuses on one's sense of well-being related to the functional effects of illness and its therapy (e.g., neuropathy related to platinum-based therapy, sexual function following oophorectomy) [16]. For example, becoming an "empty nester" may impact an individual's QOL, but that is not HRQOL. In general, QOL is impacted by a broader spectrum of factors, only one of which may be health. PROs (clinical, humanistic, and economic outcomes), including HRQOL, are important considerations to take into account when assessing the quality of cancer care.

In 2006, the U.S. Food and Drug Administration (FDA) produced its initial draft guidance for PROs, recommending the use of the term "*patient-reported outcomes*" in medical research and product development to serve as an umbrella term for all assessments, including QOL, that come directly from the patient without interpretation from clinical staff or any other person [18]. This umbrella term encompasses the broader range of self-reported assessments from the clinical symptoms a patient experiences to the more complex outcomes of care such as functional ability and quality of life. Included in the draft guidance are recommendations for selection, development and modification of PRO instruments, study design, endpoint assessment, and statistical analysis considerations [18]. Researchers should follow this guidance and refer to it in the design of clinical trials that include PROs.

11.2
Measuring Patient-Reported Outcomes (PRO)

It is estimated that nearly 200 validated PRO instruments have been created and are available, specific to physical functioning alone, and more than 200 validated instruments measure various other aspects of QOL [19, 20]. Considering that PROs can include anything that asked directly of the patient across clinical, humanistic, or economic domains, the scope is immense. The number of instruments across all these domains can be overwhelming and leads to challenges for cross-trial comparisons due to the lack of consistent use of measurement tools.

Instruments that measure PROs fall into four general categories: generic, disease-specific, dimension-specific, and utility assessments [16, 21, 22]. Generic instruments measure global constructs of well-being and can be used across diseases and dimensions. Generic instruments tend to include a broad assessment of the physical, social, and emotional domains of health and well-being [16]. They are useful for comparisons between populations and health conditions, but do not address specific issues that may be of concern in a particular diagnosis or population. The Medical Outcomes Study SF-36 Health Survey is one of the most commonly used generic PRO instruments and has been used with many different populations and diseases, including ovarian cancer [23, 24]. According to the SF-36 web site, it has been used in research reported in more than 4,000 peer-review publications and has been translated for use in more than 40 different languages and countries [25]. These translations have been reported in more than 500 peer-reviewed publications. The SF-36 includes 36 questions in eight dimensions: four dimensions of physical health (physical functioning, role-physical, bodily pain, and general health), and four dimensions of mental health (vitality, social functioning, role-emotional, and mental health), referred to as the Physical Component Survey (PCS) and Mental Component Survey (MCS), respectively. A 12-item short form (SF-12) is also available for use when cost and time are of greater concern (e.g., requires 1–2 min to complete). The SF-12 is a validated subset of the items in the SF-36 PCS and MCS [26]. Additional generic PRO instruments that have been used in cancer outcomes research are presented in Table 11.2.

Table 11.2 Selected patient-reported outcome (PRO) instruments that have been used in cancer populations

Instrument	Domains assessed
Beck depression inventory [63, 64]	Depression
Beck hopelessness scale [65, 66]	Feelings about the future Loss of motivation Future expectations
Center for epidemiologic studies depression (CES-D) scale [67, 68]	Somatic activity Depressed affect Positive affect Interpersonal affect
EuroQol 5 dimension (EQ-5D) scale[a,b] [42, 69]	Mobility Self-care Usual activities Pain/discomfort Anxiety/depression
Female sexual function index (FSFI) [70, 71]	Sexual function: desire, subjective arousal, lubrication, orgasm, satisfaction, pain
Health utilities index (HUI)[a,b] [41, 72]	HUI2: sensation, mobility, emotion, cognition, self-care, pain, fertility HUI3: vision, hearing, speech, ambulation, dexterity, emotion, cognition, pain
Hospital anxiety and depression scale (HADS) [73, 74]	Anxiety Depression
McCorkle symptom distress scale (SDS) [75, 76]	Distress related to specific symptoms: nausea, appetite, insomnia, pain, fatigue, bowel patterns, concentration, appearance, breathing, outlook
McGill quality of life questionnaire[b] [77, 78]	Physical well-being Physical symptoms Psychological well-being Existential well-being Support
Medical outcomes study short form (SF-36)[b] [23, 24, 79]	Physical function Role limitations due to physical problems Role limitations due to emotional problems Social function Emotional well-being Vitality/fatigue Pain General health perceptions

(*continued*)

Table 11.2 (continued)

Instrument	Domains assessed
Mental health inventory (MHI) [80, 81]	Anxiety Depression Positive affect Emotional ties Behavioral/emotional control
Mishel uncertainty in illness scale [82, 83]	Uncertainty in symptomatology Uncertainty in diagnosis Uncertainty in treatment Relationship with caregivers Planning for the future
Multidimensional fatigue inventory (MFI-20) [84, 85]	General fatigue Physical fatigue Mental fatigue Reduced motivation Reduced activity
Multidimensional scale of perceived social support (PSSS) [86]	Family Friends Significant others
Nottingham health profile[b] [87]	Physical mobility Pain Social isolation Emotional reactions Energy Sleep
Patient assessment of own functioning inventory (PAF) [55, 88]	Functional abilities in five categories: memory, language/communication, use of hands, sensory/perceptual, cognitive/intellectual
Profile of mood states (POMS) [89, 90]	Tension-anxiety Depression-dejection Anger-hostility Vigor-activity Fatigue-inertia Confusion-bewilderment
Quality of well-being scale (QWB-SA)[b] [91–93]	Symptoms/problem complex Mobility Physical activity Self-care/social role activity
Rotterdam symptom checklist[b] [8, 94, 95]	Physical symptom distress Psychological distress Activity level Overall QOL
Sickness impact profile (SIP)[b] [96, 97]	Physical: ambulation, mobility, body care, movement Psychosocial: social interaction, communication, alertness behavior, emotional behavior, sleep and rest, eating, home management, recreation and pastimes, employment

Table 11.2 (continued)

Instrument	Domains assessed
Spielberger state-trait anxiety inventory (STAI) [98, 99]	Anxiety
World Health Organization quality of life-100 (WHOQOL-100)[b] [100, 101]	Physical Psychological Level of independence Social relationships Environment Spirituality/religion/beliefs Overall QOL

[a]Utility measure
[b]Generic instrument

Disease-specific instruments are those that were developed and validated in a population with a particular condition and may assess several domains that are relevant to those who have experienced that condition. Table 11.3 presents a number of instruments that have been developed and validated specifically for use in cancer populations. Currently, the majority of PRO instruments that have been developed for cancer populations have focused on physical functioning and global QOL assessments. Some of the frequently used disease-specific instruments include the functional assessment of cancer therapy (FACT), the European Organization for Research and Treatment of Cancer (EORTC) quality of life questionnaire (QLQ-30), and the functional living index-cancer (FLIC) [22]. The FACT-G can be used among patients with any cancer diagnosis, regardless of the treatment received.

Table 11.3 Selected PRO instruments designed specifically for cancer populations

Instrument	Domains assessed
Cancer rehabilitation evaluation system (CARES) [102]	Physical Psychosocial Medical interaction/communication Marital Sexual
EORTC ovarian cancer module (EORTC QLQ-OV28) [29, 66][a]	Abdominal/gastrointestinal symptoms Peripheral neuropathy Other chemotherapy side effects Hormonal/menopausal symptoms Body image Attitude to disease/treatment Sexual functioning
EORTC quality of life questionnaire (QLQ-30) [103][b]	Physical functioning Role functioning Cognitive functioning Emotional functioning Social functioning Global health status/QOL Fatigue Nausea/vomiting Miscellaneous concerns (e.g., sleep, finances)

(continued)

Table 11.3 (continued)

Instrument	Domains assessed
Ferrans and powers quality of life index-cancer version [104–106]	Health and physical Socioeconomic Psychological and spiritual Family
Fox simple quality of life scale (FSQOLS) [107]	Physical Psychological Social Spiritual QOL (health, well-being, functioning, satisfaction)
Functional assessment of cancer therapy for ovarian cancer (FACT-O) [28][a]	FACT-G: Physical, social/family, emotional, functional well-being Additional concerns of ovarian cancer

Functional assessment of cancer therapy (FACT) – symptom/treatment subscales [27][b]	Subscales available for:
	  Neurotoxicity
	  Anorexia/cachexia
	  Anemia/fatigue
	  Bone pain
	  Lymphedema
	  Incontinence (urinary/fecal)
	  Neutropenia
	  Thrombocytopenia
	  Palliative care
	  Taxane treatment
	  Treatment satisfaction
	  Spirituality

Functional living index-cancer (FLIC) [34, 108]	Physical Psychological Social functioning Nausea Hardship due to cancer Overall QOL (well-being)
Functional living index-emesis [109, 110]	Nausea Vomiting
Global quality of life scale (GLQ-8/GLQ uniscale) [111]	Anxiety/depression Nausea/vomiting Numbness Loss of hair Tiredness Appetite/taste Sexuality Thoughts about treatment
Impact of cancer (IOC) scale [112]	Positive impact: altruism/empathy, health awareness, meaning of cancer, positive self-evaluation Negative impact: appearance concerns, body change concerns, life interferences, worry Employment concerns Relationship concerns

Table 11.3 (continued)

Instrument	Domains assessed
Individualized quality of life scale [113, 114]	Satisfaction (with 14 areas of life) Importance (of those 14 areas of life)
M.D. Anderson symptom inventory (MDASI) [115]	General symptoms: pain, fatigue, disturbed sleep, emotional distress, shortness of breath, drowsiness, dry mouth, sadness, remembering, numbness/tingling Gastrointestinal symptoms: nausea, emesis
Memorial symptom assessment scale (MSAS) [116]	Psychological symptoms: sadness, worry, irritability, nervousness, sleep, concentration Physical symptoms: appetite, energy, pain, drowsiness, constipation, dry mouth, nausea, vomiting, change in taste, weight loss, bloating, dizziness Distress
Northouse fear of recurrence (FOR) questionnaire [66, 117]	Concerns of disease recurrence
Patient assessment, care, and education (PACE) system [118]	Computerized, tablet-based system for collection of chemotherapy-related symptoms
Quality of life index (QLI) [119]	Psychological Physical Symptoms Financial protection
Quality of life survey for cancer [120]	Physical Psychological Symptom control Social support/social concerns
Social difficulties inventory (SDI) [121]	Social distress
Spitzer quality of life index (QL-index) [49][c]	Activity (own occupation) Activities of daily living General health Social support Outlook on life

[a]Developed specifically for ovarian cancer

[b]Additional domain-specific and other disease site-specific instruments are available

[c]Although can be administered as a PRO instrument, traditionally is completed by the health care provider and was not developed to measure PRO

The FACT-G is a 27-item scale measuring patient-reported QOL specifically related to cancer [27] and includes four subscales: physical well-being, functional well-being, social well-being, and emotional well-being. Each item is scored from 0 to 4, with total scores that may range from 0 to 108. While the FACT-G is a disease-specific instrument designed for use in cancer, it enables data collection across cancer sites and can be completed in a brief encounter in the clinic. The FACT-O is an ovarian cancer-specific instrument that includes the FACT-G plus a subscale specific to concerns of women with ovarian cancer. These concerns include abdominal swelling, vomiting, appetite, bowel function, hair loss, body appearance, mobility, sexual function, fertility and abdominal cramping, and body weight [28]. The FACT-O has been shown to correlate with the FLIC in an ovarian cancer patient population, with the exception of the social well-being domain [28].

The EORTC QLQ-30 was developed in the early 1990s to measure global QOL and outcomes in the five domains of physical, emotional, social, cognitive, and role functioning. The QLQ-30 also measures symptoms (fatigue, nausea/vomiting, and pain) and contains items that assess dyspnea, sleep issues, appetite, constipation, diarrhea, and the financial impact of care [29]. It was developed specifically to assess the well-being of individuals enrolled in clinical trials as a means of standardizing outcomes across studies [30]. The EORTC QLQ-30 is similar to the FACT instruments in that they both have additional supplementary modules to assess specific disease sites (e.g., ovarian cancer) and other outcomes (e.g., pain, satisfaction, palliative care). It has been validated in more than 60 languages worldwide and is used extensively in cancer research. Despite their similarities, the domains assessed by the EORTC QLQ-C30 and FACT-G are not directly comparable. A study comparing these tools found little agreement on all domains with the exception of physical functioning ($r = 0.66$) [31]. Since the domains of well-being are very broad (e.g., social, emotional), this is not surprising, but is a reminder to use caution while making cross-trial comparisons of PROs that use different instruments for the same underlying construct. The minimally important difference of EORTC QLQ-C30 scores have been published and manuals are available from the EORTC, which provide detailed guidance on the determination of sample size and power for outcomes assessment using this instrument [32]. The EORTC QLQ-OV28 (OV28) is a disease-specific instrument that was developed and validated specifically for PROs in ovarian cancer populations [29, 33]. The items in the OV28 include abdominal/gastrointestinal symptoms, peripheral neuropathy, other chemotherapy side effects, hormonal/menopausal symptoms, body image, attitude to disease/treatment, and sexual functioning. The items included in this subscale were initially developed by culling the literature, expert panel consideration of factors, and review by ovarian cancer patients and were finalized through a series of psychometric studies [29, 33].

The FLIC was developed in the 1980s as one of the earliest disease-specific instruments to assess cancer-related PROs [30, 34]. The FLIC focuses on functional ability and the impact of cancer on daily activities across several domains (physical, psychological, social functioning, hardship due to cancer, overall well-being, and concerns specific to nausea). It was developed to be reliable for longitudinal assessment and to have sufficient sensitivity to concerns so that populations could be compared, specifically in clinical trial settings [34, 35]. It has been shown to have similar sensitivity as the QLQ-30 and greater sensitivity than other generic instruments [36, 37]. Initial items were developed based on a literature review, patient interviews, and a panel consisting of patients, caregivers, and clergy. The items were then reduced via a series of psychometric studies and were validated against other standard assessments (e.g., Katz activities of daily living index, Beck depression scale, Speilberger state-trait anxiety scale, and others) [34]. The FLIC provides a total summary score, ranging from 22 to 154, which reflects overall quality of life, with higher scores representing greater quality of life.

Domain-specific instruments address a specific aspect of well-being (e.g., sexual function, depression) and are not designed to measure the broader scope of QOL or well-being.

Domain-specific measures may also be disease-specific, such as the functional living index-emesis that measures the patient experience related to the nausea and vomiting during cancer treatment, or may be used across conditions, such as the Beck depression inventory. There are hundreds of instruments that have been designed to assess many different specific aspects of health outcomes, and new instruments are being published on a regular basis. All new instruments must undergo thorough development and refinement procedures, followed by psychometric evaluation and validation in the target population before they are ready to be implemented for outcomes research [38]. Therefore, it is prudent to conduct a thorough literature review to identify existing validated instruments that may target the underlying constructs of interest prior to beginning the process of developing a new survey. Examples of several validated domain-specific instruments that have been designed specifically for cancer are included in Table 11.3, and those that can be used across conditions, including cancer, are included in Table 11.2.

Utility instruments differ in their focus, in that they have been developed specifically for use in health economic analyses. Utility instruments provide a single health status score for each respondent. These scores can be associated with a preference value that has been determined through population-based studies. Preference values range from 0.0 to 1.0, representing anchors of death and perfect health, respectively. These preference scores associated with utility instruments are thought to reflect population-based values of the health state. These values can then be used to adjust outcomes of care to estimate quality-adjusted life years (QALYs) in economic analyses. QALYs incorporate both quantity and QOL in one score [21, 39]. For example, the population-based preference value of a health condition may be 0.75. If a person was expected to survive 5 years in that health condition, this would equal to 3.75 QALYs (5 years × value of 0.75). This could be compared to any other heath condition that was also adjusted for quantity and quality of life, or to perfect health for that same time period (5.0 QALYs-5 years × value of perfect health, 1.0). Several generic instruments are available that have been associated with preference values, such as the EuroQol 5 dimension (EQ-5D) scale, health utilities index (HUI), and the short form 6 dimension utility index (SF-6D), which is calculated from a subset of items from the SF-36 [40–42]. These instruments are described in more detail below. In addition to instruments that have been used to measure utilities, methods have been used that calculate quality-adjusted time without symptoms of disease or toxicity of treatment (Q-TWiST), to estimate an overall benefit of treatment that incorporates survival, progression, and toxicities [43]. Instead of relying on population-based estimates of the value of a health condition, treatment outcomes are weighted in terms of the toxicity (severity and duration of side effects) and survival (time spent disease-free and overall survival). TWiST is calculated as the disease-free survival time (DFS) minus the time during which a patient experiences the toxic side effects of therapy. TWiST is then adjusted for quality (Q-TWiST) by calculating the utility coefficients for various periods during the overall survival time [43]. This method has been applied to a cost-effectiveness analysis of IV paclitaxel for the front-line treatment of ovarian cancer, but is not known to have been used in the setting of intraperitoneal (IP) treatment [44].

As PROs are increasingly becoming the focus of medical care, additional instruments are being developed or are being adapted from other settings that take a broader approach to the clinical, humanistic, and economic outcomes of cancer care (e.g., satisfaction with care, cognitive function, communication with providers, the economic impact of illness).

There is a need for the consistent use of reliable, validated outcomes assessment instruments that capture aspects of humanistic, clinical, and economic outcomes of cancer care. The National Institutes of Health developed the Patient-Reported Outcomes Measurement Information System (PROMIS) initiative to create a data bank of PRO items from existing, validated questionnaires [45, 46]. The goals of this collaborative effort are to improve PRO assessment across chronic diseases by providing an electronic, publicly available repository of validated items and to provide investigators with surveys that can be customized to enhance cross-trial comparisons.

11.3
Quality of Life and Patient-Reported Outcomes of Intraperitoneal Therapy

In 1986, the Southwest Oncology Group (SWOG) activated protocol number 8501, the first of several large, phase III trials investigating IP cisplatin for the front-line treatment of advanced ovarian cancer [47]. Five hundred and forty-six (546) eligible patients were included in the final analysis. Patients were randomized to either intravenous (IV) or IP therapy. Both the IV and IP groups received 600 mg/m² cyclophosophamide plus 100 mg/m² cisplatin on day 1 of every 21 days for six cycles. The groups only differed on the mode of administration of the cisplatin: 279 were randomized to receive IV cisplatin and 267 were randomized to receive IP cisplatin. Completion of treatment was equivalent between both groups, with 58% of patients in both groups completing the full six courses of chemotherapy. In this study, there were significantly higher granulocytopenia, leukopenia, and neuromuscular toxicities in the IV group. The IP group experienced greater ototoxicity and there were two treatment-related deaths [47]. Survival was significantly greater among those receiving IP therapy (hazard ratio [HR] = 0.76; 95% confidence interval [95% CI], 0.61–0.96; p = 0.02) [47]. One hundred and sixty-nine women (87 and 82 randomized to the IV and IP group, respectively) were included in an interim QOL analysis of SWOG 8501 [48].

QOL was assessed in SWOG 8501 by the QL-index at each of the six cycles of treatment. The QL-index was developed as a tool for physicians to record patient QOL in the categories of activity, daily living, health, support, and outlook on life [49]. Performance status, measured by the Eastern Cooperative Oncology Group (ECOG) performance status scale [50], and adverse events were also collected each cycle and analyzed specifically for this analysis. Among patients randomized to IV therapy in SWOG 8501, there were significantly higher scores in the categories of activity (cycles 3, 4, and 5), daily living (cycles 4, 5, and 6), and outlook (cycles 1, 4, and 5) [48]. Differences in QL-index scores were in the range of 0.2–0.3 between groups out of the total possible range of 0.0–10.0, so although statistically significant, the differences were small. QOL increased in both groups over the course of treatment (from cycle 1 through cycle 6; p = 0.001). Although ECOG performance status was equivalent over time in both groups (p = 0.932), those treated with IP therapy had lower overall QOL assessments as measured by the QL-index over the course of treatment (p = 0.0008) [48]. QOL was significantly correlated with toxicity (p < 0.001); this relationship was consistent between the activities, daily living, and outlook categories, but was not related to social support [48]. When individual toxicities were assessed, abdominal cramping (cycles 2 and 3 only), constipation (cycle 6), and abdominal pain (cycles 2 and 5 only) were higher among those treated with IP therapy. Cystitis/bladder toxicity (cycle 6) was higher among those treated with IV therapy. All patients lost weight during treatment ($p = 0.001$) [48]. Patients receiving IP therapy were reported to experience periodic lower reported QOL in activities (daily and occupational) and outlook on life during treatment, but these differences did not persist over time (e.g., self-reported activities and outlook were equivalent between the IV and IP treatment groups by cycle 6 of treatment). This study was limited by a small sample size, but suggests that the differential impact on QOL of IP therapy as compared to IV treatment may be short lived.

Unfortunately, this study only collected physician-reported quality of life of the patient and did not elicit the patient's perspective on their own QOL. Instruments such as the QL-index have been shown to correlate with patient self-ratings ($p = 0.61–0.69$) and to show strong correlation between independent physician assessments ($p = 0.74–0.84$) [49]. SWOG 8501 may have been the first to have routinely collected QOL data related to IP therapy and to demonstrate a direct relationship between toxicity and QOL in the IP setting, but is limited by the lack of PRO. The best source of data about how the patient is feeling on therapy is the patient herself.

The Gynecologic Oncology Group (GOG) initiated a randomized trial of IP chemotherapy to follow the findings of prior GOG and SWOG studies. In this study (protocol GOG 0172), 415 eligible study participants were randomized to either receive IV therapy (135 mg/m^2 paclitaxel over 24-h IV on day 1 followed by 75 mg/m^2 cisplatin IV on day 2) or IP therapy (135 mg/m^2 paclitaxel over 24-h IV on day 1, 100 mg/m^2 cisplatin IP on day 2, followed by 60 mg/m^2 paclitaxel IP on day 8) [51]. Eighty-three percent (83%) of the 210 patients randomized to IV therapy completed all six cycles of the assigned study treatment and 42% of the 205 eligible patients randomized to IP therapy completed all six cycles of the assigned study treatment. Patients randomized to IP therapy experienced greater serious adverse events (grade 3 and 4), including greater pain, fatigue, and hematologic, gastrointestinal, metabolic, and neurologic toxicities as compared to those randomized to IV therapy ($p < 0.001$). Patients randomized to IP therapy had greater progression-free (23.8 months IP vs. 18.3 months IV, $p = 0.05$) and overall survival (65.6 months IP vs. 49.7 months IV, $p = 0.03$) [51].

QOL and patient-reported neuropathy outcomes were assessed in GOG 0172 using the FACT-O (general cancer and ovarian-specific scales) and the FACT-Ntx (neuropathy subscale) [52]. Two additional items were added to the FACT scales to assess patient-reported abdominal discomfort. PRO assessments were completed prior to randomization, prior to cycle 4, approximately 1 month after completing treatment, and 12 months after treatment. Of the 415 patients eligible for assessment, 54% completed all four assessments, with significantly fewer patients in the IP group completing all assessments as compared to those in the IV group. Prior to randomization, patients who later received IP therapy had significantly lower QOL than those who received IV therapy on all QOL scales (FACT-G, $p = 0.02$; FACT-O, $p = 0.007$) and on the abdominal discomfort assessment ($p = 0.05$). There remained a significant difference in all PROs throughout the treatment period, even after controlling for baseline differences in FACT scores between groups, with the exception of abdominal discomfort, which was equivalent between the IP and IV groups as soon as one month post-treatment [51, 52]. One year after the completion of treatment, both groups reported equivalent QOL ($p>0.70$) and equivalent abdominal discomfort ($p=0.93$). The IP group continued to report greater neuropathy one year postcompletion of treatment ($p=0.003$) [52]. Although the completion rates were low (54%) and there were differential completion rates between groups ($p=0.035$), this study does provide initial evidence suggesting the lack of long-term negative effects on QOL following IP therapy. It also suggests that neuropathy may be an increased long-term concern for patients receiving high doses of IP therapy. Persistent neuropathy was reported in GOG 0172 where there was a higher dose of cisplatin given to patients receiving IP therapy (e.g., 100 mg/m^2 cisplatin on the IP arm vs. 75 mg/m^2 cisplatin on the IV arm) [51]; however, there were no differences in neuropathy in SWOG 8501, where both the IP and IV groups received 100 mg/m^2 cisplatin [47].

Unfortunately, other than physician-reported QOL data from the QL-index in SWOG 8501 and the PRO from the FACT scales in GOG 0172, very little humanistic PRO data have been collected related to IP therapy in the front-line setting of advanced ovarian cancer. The perceived impact of IP therapy on the patient is one important reason for the lack of implementation of IP therapy in the front-line setting [53]. However, PROs have been consistently lacking in the studies of this treatment modality, and much is left to assumption or opinion. This lack points to the critical need to include well-designed PRO components in any clinical trial. The lack of this information may impact the adoption rate of new treatments and reduce controversy over new methods of treatment. While clinical outcomes data provide strong evidence for the benefits of IP therapy, these outcomes continue to be debated [54, 55]. This debate is encouraged and sustained by the lack of scientific information about the humanistic outcomes of IP therapy. Perhaps, with sufficient PRO data from future trials and the development and implementation of interventions to reduce any adverse impact on humanistic and clinical outcomes, the current viable options for the treatment of newly diagnosed, advanced ovarian cancer may become more widely accepted [56, 57].

While PROs have not routinely been collected for the front-line IP treatment of ovarian cancer, some studies that have assessed second-line IP therapy have included PRO [58]. Although second-line therapy studies have not shown any differences in QOL among patients treated with IP as compared to IV administration, the sample sizes have been small and likely not sufficiently powered to be able to detect any differences. Although all studies of IP therapy have included toxicity assessments, usually using the NCI common toxicity criteria (CTC), toxicity data are not QOL data, and toxicity as recorded by the CTC is not necessarily a PRO. However, there does tend to be an inverse relationship between toxicity and QOL and other PROs. In research of ovarian cancer treatment modalities, there is a need to expand assessments to include the perspective of the patient. The experience of IP treatment can be better understood if the patient's point of view is considered. Toxicity assessments are, at best, a rough estimation of how the patient is feeling in the broader domains of well-being.

While IP therapy has been shown to improve survival [51, 59], the primary reason for the lack of incorporation of the regimen in routine practice was due to concerns about toxicity (specifically neurologic toxicity, gastrointestinal toxicity, catheter infection, and nephropathy) [53]. While editorials and reviews of physician perspectives on the pros and cons of IP therapy are widely available [60–62], the patient perspective during treatment with IP therapy is greatly lacking and is clearly needed [54]. What is known, however, is that women who receive IP therapy live significantly longer, and although there is an initial impact on quality of life, these effects are not long term.

11.4
Conclusion

To fully understand the value and impact of care, data must be collected that measure patients' perspectives of their own well-being. The selection of PRO instruments must take into account the type of outcome that is of interest (e.g., clinical, economic, or humanistic). Many validated generic, disease- and domain-specific instruments are available that can provide information on overall well-being, as well as on the impact of treatment on many specific aspects of individual quality of life, health outcomes, and social/interpersonal relationships. The selection of instruments should take into account the anticipated impact of the treatment as well as the research question that is being asked. In the setting of IP therapy, there are many unanswered questions due to the lack of data collected from the patients' perspective. It is critical that this information be incorporated into future research efforts that utilize IP regimens, so that some of the debate can be resolved regarding the impact of this treatment on the patient.

References

1. WHO. Preamble to the Constitution of the World Health Organization as adopted by the International Health Conference, New York, 19–22 June 1946; signed on 22 July 1946 by the representatives of 61 States (Official Records of the World Health Organization, no 2, p 100) and entered into force on 7 April 1948
2. Lipscomb J, Donaldson MS, Arora NK, Brown ML, Clauser SB, Potosky AL et al (2004) Cancer outcomes research. J Natl Cancer Inst monographs (33):178–197
3. Goodman MT, Correa CN, Tung KH, Roffers SD, Cheng Wu X, Young JL Jr et al (2003) Stage at diagnosis of ovarian cancer in the United States, 1992–1997. Cancer 97(10 suppl):2648–2659
4. Krouse R, Aziz NM (2008) Cancer survivorship. In: Alberts DS, Hess LM (eds) Fundamentals of cancer prevention. Springer, Heidelberg
5. Ferrell B, Smith SL, Cullinane CA, Melancon C (2003) Psychological well being and quality of life in ovarian cancer survivors. Cancer 98(5):1061–1071
6. Ferrell BR, Smith SL, Ervin KS, Itano J, Melancon C (2003) A qualitative analysis of social concerns of women with ovarian cancer. Psycho-oncology 12(7):647–663
7. Houck K, Avis NE, Gallant JM, Fuller AF Jr, Goodman A (1999) Quality of life in advanced ovarian cancer: identifying specific concerns. J Palliat Med 2(4):397–402
8. Montazeri A, McEwen J, Gillis CR (1996) Quality of life in patients with ovarian cancer: current state of research. Support Care Cancer 4(3):169–179
9. Sun CC, Bodurka DC, Weaver CB, Rasu R, Wolf JK, Bevers MW et al (2005) Rankings and symptom assessments of side effects from chemotherapy: insights from experienced patients with ovarian cancer. Support Care Cancer 13(4):219–227
10. IOM (2008) Cancer care for the whole patient. National Academy Press, Washington, DC
11. Passik SD, Kirsh KL (2005) A pilot examination of the impact of cancer patients' fatigue on their spousal caregivers. Palliat Support Care 3(4):273–279
12. Awadalla AW, Ohaeri JU, Gholoum A, Khalid AO, Hamad HM, Jacob A (2007) Factors associated with quality of life of outpatients with breast cancer and gynecologic cancers and their family caregivers: a controlled study. BMC Cancer 7:102

13. Le T, Leis A, Pahwa P, Wright K, Ali K, Reeder B (2003) Quality-of-life issues in patients with ovarian cancer and their caregivers: a review. Obstet Gynecol Surv 58(11):749–758

14. Ponto JA, Barton D (2008) Husbands' perspective of living with wives' ovarian cancer. Psycho-oncology 17(12):1225–1231

15. Donabedian A (1980) The definition of quality: a conceptual exploration. Explorations in quality assessment and monitoring. Health Administration Press, Ann Arbor

16. Berzon RA, Lobo FS (2006) Measuring health-related quality of life within clinical research studies. In: Chumney ECG, Simpson KN (eds) Methods and designs for outcomes research. American Society of Health-System Pharmacists, Bethesda, MD

17. Bond J, Corner L (2004) Explaining quality of life. In: Corner L (ed) Quality of life and older people. Open University Press, Maidenhead

18. FDA (2006) Patient-reported outcome measures: use in medical product development to support labeling claims [cited June 15, 2009]. http://www.fda.gov/downloads/Drugs/GuidanceCompliance RegulatoryInformation/Guidances/UCM071975.pdf

19. Fries JF, Krishnan E, Bruce B (2009) Items, instruments, crosswalks, and PROMIS. J Rheumatol 36(6):1093–1095

20. Salek S (1999) Compendium of quality of life instruments. Chichester, Wiley

21. Coons SJ, Craig BM (2008) Assessing human and economic benefits of cancer prevention. In: Alberts DS, Hess LM (eds) Fundamentals of cancer prevention. Springer, Heidelberg

22. Garratt A, Schmidt L, Mackintosh A, Fitzpatrick R (2002) Quality of life measurement: bibliographic study of patient assessed health outcome measures. BMJ 324(7351):1417

23. Gil KM, Gibbons HE, Jenison EL, Hopkins MP, von Gruenigen VE (2007) Baseline characteristics influencing quality of life in women undergoing gynecologic oncology surgery. Health Qual Life Outcomes 5:25

24. von Gruenigen VE, Frasure HE, Jenison EL, Hopkins MP, Gil KM (2006) Longitudinal assessment of quality of life and lifestyle in newly diagnosed ovarian cancer patients: the roles of surgery and chemotherapy. Gynecol Oncol 103(1):120–126

25. Ware JE (2009) SF-35 health survey update [cited June 29, 2009]. http://www.sf-36.org/tools/sf36.shtml

26. Ware JE, Kosinski M, Keller SD (1996) A 12-item short-form health survey: construction of scales and preliminary tests of reliability and validity. Med Care 34(3):220–233

27. Cella DF, Tulsky DS, Gray G, Sarafian B, Linn E, Bonomi A et al (1993) The functional assessment of cancer therapy scale: development and validation of the general measure. J Clin Oncol 11(3):570–579

28. Basen-Engquist K, Bodurka-Bevers D, Fitzgerald MA, Webster K, Cella D, Hu S et al (2001) Reliability and validity of the functional assessment of cancer therapy-ovarian. J Clin Oncol 19(6): 1809–1817

29. Greimel E, Bottomley A, Cull A, Waldenstrom AC, Arraras J, Chauvenet L et al (2003) An international field study of the reliability and validity of a disease-specific questionnaire module (the QLQ-OV28) in assessing the quality of life of patients with ovarian cancer. Eur J Cancer 39(10):1402–1408

30. Bonomi AE, Shikiar R, Legro MW (2000) Quality-of-life assessment in acute, chronic, and cancer pain: a pharmacist's guide. J Am Pharm Assoc 40(3):402–416

31. Kemmler G, Holzner B, Kopp M, Dunser M, Margreiter R, Greil R et al (1999) Comparison of two quality-of-life instruments for cancer patients: the functional assessment of cancer therapy-general and the European Organization for Research and Treatment of Cancer Quality of Life Questionnaire-C30. J Clin Oncol 17(9):2932–2940

32. King MT (1996) The interpretation of scores from the EORTC quality of life questionnaire QLQ-C30. Qual Life Res 5(6):555–567

33. Cull A, Howat S, Greimel E, Waldenstrom AC, Arraras J, Kudelka A et al (2001) Development of a European organization for research and treatment of cancer questionnaire module to

assess the quality of life of ovarian cancer patients in clinical trials: a progress report. Eur J Cancer 37(1):47–53

34. Schipper H, Clinch J, McMurray A, Levitt M (1984) Measuring the quality of life of cancer patients: the functional living index-cancer: development and validation. J Clin Oncol 2(5): 472–483

35. Finkelstein DM, Cassileth BR, Bonomi PD, Ruckdeschel JC, Ezdinli EZ, Wolter JM (1988) A pilot study of the functional living index-cancer (FLIC) Scale for the assessment of quality of life for metastatic lung cancer patients. An Eastern Cooperative Oncology Group study. Am J Clin Oncol 11(6):630–633

36. King M (1999) Responsiveness of the functional living index-cancer (FLIC) and the EORTC core quality of life (QOL) module (QLQ-C30). Qual Life Res 8(7):610

37. Wilson RW, Hutson LM, Vanstry D (2005) Comparison of 2 quality-of-life questionnaires in women treated for breast cancer: the RAND 36-item health survey and the functional living index-cancer. Phys Ther 85(9):851–860

38. Turner RR, Quittner AL, Parasuraman BM, Kallich JD, Cleeland CS, Mayo/FDA Patient-Reported Outcomes Consensus Meeting Group (2007) Patient-reported outcomes: instrument development and selection issues. Value Health 10(suppl 2):S86–S93

39. Mauskopf J (2006) Utility assessment. In: Chumney ECG, Simpson KN (eds) Methods and designs for outcomes research. American Society of Health-System Pharmacists, Inc., Bethesda, MD

40. Brazier J, Roberts J, Deverill M (2002) The estimation of a preference-based measure of health from the SF-36. J Health Econ 21(2):271–292

41. Horsman J, Furlong W, Feeny D, Torrance G (2003) The health utilities index (HUI): concepts, measurement properties and applications. Health Qual Life Outcomes 1:54

42. Pickard AS, Wilke CT, Lin HW, Lloyd A (2007) Health utilities using the EQ-5D in studies of cancer. Pharmacoeconomics 25(5):365–384

43. Gelber RD, Goldhirsch A, Cole BF, International Breast Cancer Study Group (1993) Evaluation of effectiveness: Q-TWiST. Cancer Treat Rev 19(suppl A):73–84

44. Limat S, Woronoff-Lemsi MC, Menat C, Madroszyk-Flandin A, Merrouche Y (2004) From randomised clinical trials to clinical practice: a pragmatic cost-effectiveness analysis of paclitaxel in first-line therapy for advanced ovarian cancer. Pharmacoeconomics 22(10):633–641

45. Garcia SF, Cella D, Clauser SB, Flynn KE, Lad T, Lai JS et al (2007) Standardizing patient-reported outcomes assessment in cancer clinical trials: a patient-reported outcomes measurement information system initiative. J Clin Oncol 25(32):5106–5112

46. Rose M, Bjorner JB, Becker J, Fries JF, Ware JE (2008) Evaluation of a preliminary physical function item bank supported the expected advantages of the patient-reported outcomes measurement information system (PROMIS). J Clin Epidemiol 61(1):17–33

47. Alberts DS, Liu PY, Hannigan EV, O'Toole R, Williams SD, Young JA et al (1996) Intraperitoneal cisplatin plus intravenous cyclophosphamide versus intravenous cisplatin plus intravenous cyclophosphamide for stage III ovarian cancer. N Engl J Med 335(26):1950–1955

48. Davis AL (1991) Adverse effects and quality of life estimates in women receiving intravenous vs intraperitoneal chemotherapy for stage III ovarian cancer. University of Washington, Takoma, Dissertation.

49. Spitzer WO, Dobson AJ, Hall J, Chesterman E, Levi J, Shepherd R et al (1981) Measuring the quality of life of cancer patients: a concise QL-index for use by physicians. J Chronic Dis 34(12): 585–597

50. Oken MM, Creech RH, Tormey DC, Horton J, Davis TE, McFadden ET, Carbone PP (1982) Toxicity and response criteria of the Eastern Cooperative Oncology Group. Am J Clin Oncol 5: 649–655

51. Armstrong DK, Bundy B, Wenzel L, Huang HQ, Baergen R, Lele S et al (2006) Intraperitoneal cisplatin and paclitaxel in ovarian cancer. N Engl J Med 354(1):34–43

52. Wenzel LB, Huang HQ, Armstrong DK, Walker JL, Cella D (2007) Health-related quality of life during and after intraperitoneal versus intravenous chemotherapy for optimally debulked ovarian cancer: a Gynecologic Oncology Group Study. J Clin Oncol 25(4):437–443

53. Naumann RW, Sukumvanich P, Edwards RP (2009) Practice patterns of intraperitoneal chemotherapy in women with ovarian cancer. Gynecol Oncol 114(1):37–41

54. Hess LM, Alberts DS (2007) The role of intraperitoneal therapy in advanced ovarian cancer. Oncology 21(2):227–232; discussion 32, 35, 39–42

55. Hess LM, Chambers SK, Hallum A, Janicek M, Buscema J, Slayton L, Chongpison Y, Calley C, Alberts DS (2010) Pilot study of the identification of changes in cognitive function in ovarian cancer patients. submitted

56. ACOG Committee Opinion No. 396 (2008) Intraperitoneal chemotherapy for ovarian cancer. Obstet Gynecol 111(1):249

57. Trimble EL, Christian MC (2008) National Cancer Institute-United States strategy regarding intraperitoneal chemotherapy for ovarian cancer. Int J Gynecol Cancer 18(suppl 1):26–28

58. Majdak E, Krasinska L, Mielcarek P, Kobierski J, Kozaka J, Milczek T et al (2002) Comparison of quality of life in patients with advanced ovarian cancer treated with intraperitoneal or intravenous cisplatin and cyclophosphamide as a second line of therapy. Ginekol Pol 73(11): 1096–1102

59. Hess LM, Benham-Hutchins M, Herzog TJ, Hsu CH, Malone DC, Skrepnek GH et al (2007) A meta-analysis of the efficacy of intraperitoneal cisplatin for the front-line treatment of ovarian cancer. Int J Gynecol Cancer 17(3):561–570

60. Alberts DS, Markman M, Muggia F, Ozols RF, Eldermire E, Bookman MA et al (2006) Proceedings of a GOG workshop on intraperitoneal therapy for ovarian cancer. Gynecol Oncol 103(3):783–792

61. Armstrong DK, Brady MF (2006) Intraperitoneal therapy for ovarian cancer: a treatment ready for prime time. J Clin Oncol 24(28):4531–4533

62. Vergote I, Amant F, Leunen K, Cadron I, Van Gorp T, Neven P et al (2008) Intraperitoneal chemotherapy in patients with advanced ovarian cancer: the con view. Oncologist 13(4): 410–414

63. Beck AT, Steer RA (1984) Internal consistencies of the original and revised beck depression inventory. J Clin Psychol 40(6):1365–1367

64. Norton TR, Manne SL, Rubin S, Carlson J, Hernandez E, Edelson MI et al (2004) Prevalence and predictors of psychological distress among women with ovarian cancer. J Clin Oncol 22(5): 919–926

65. Beck AT, Weissman A, Lester D, Trexler L (1974) The measurement of pessimism: the hopelessness scale. J Consult Clin Psychol 42(6):861–865

66. Mirabeau-Beale KL, Kornblith AB, Penson RT, Lee H, Goodman A, Campos SM et al (2009) Comparison of the quality of life of early and advanced stage ovarian cancer survivors. Gynecol Oncol 114(2):353–359

67. Hann D, Winter K, Jacobsen P (1999) Measurement of depressive symptoms in cancer patients: evaluation of the Center for Epidemiological Studies Depression Scale (CES-D). J Psychosom Res 46(5):437–443

68. van Wilgen CP, Dijkstra PU, Stewart RE, Ranchor AV, Roodenburg JL (2006) Measuring somatic symptoms with the CES-D to assess depression in cancer patients after treatment: comparison among patients with oral/oropharyngeal, gynecological, colorectal, and breast cancer. Psychosomatics 47(6):465–470

69. Szende A, Oppe M, Devlin N (2007) EQ-5D value sets. Springer, Dordrecht

70. Carter J, Rowland K, Chi D, Brown C, Abu-Rustum N, Castiel M et al (2005) Gynecologic cancer treatment and the impact of cancer-related infertility. Gynecol Oncol 97(1):90–95

71. Rosen R, Brown C, Heiman J, Leiblum S, Meston C, Shabsigh R et al (2000) The female sexual function index (FSFI): a multidimensional self-report instrument for the assessment of female sexual function. J Sex Marital Ther 26(2):191–208

72. Whitton AC, Rhydderch H, Furlong W, Feeny D, Barr RD (1997) Self-reported comprehensive health status of adult brain tumor patients using the health utilities index. Cancer 80(2): 258–265

73. Price MA, Zachariae R, Butow PN, Defazio A, Chauhan D, Espie CA et al (2009) Prevalence and predictors of insomnia in women with invasive ovarian cancer: anxiety a major factor. Eur J Cancer 45(18):3262–70.

74. Zigmond AS, Snaith RP (1983) The hospital anxiety and depression scale. Acta Psychiatr Scand 67(6):361–370

75. McCorkle R, Quint-Benoliel J (1983) Symptom distress, current concerns and mood disturbance after diagnosis of life-threatening disease. Soc Sci Med 17(7):431–438

76. McCorkle R, Dowd M, Ercolano E, Schulman-Green D, Williams AL, Siefert ML et al (2009) Effects of a nursing intervention on quality of life outcomes in post-surgical women with gynecological cancers. Psychooncology 18(1):62–70

77. Cohen SR, Mount BM (2000) Living with cancer: "good" days and "bad" days – what produces them? Can the McGill quality of life questionnaire distinguish between them? Cancer 89(8): 1854–1865

78. Cohen SR, Mount BM, Strobel MG, Bui F (1995) The McGill quality of life questionnaire: a measure of quality of life appropriate for people with advanced disease. A preliminary study of validity and acceptability. Palliat Med 9(3):207–219

79. Cooley ME, McCorkle R, Knafl GJ, Rimar J, Barbieri MJ, Davies M et al (2005) Comparison of health-related quality of life questionnaires in ambulatory oncology. Qual Life Res 14(5): 1239–1249

80. Norton TR, Manne SL, Rubin S, Hernandez E, Carlson J, Bergman C et al (2005) Ovarian cancer patients' psychological distress: the role of physical impairment, perceived unsupportive family and friend behaviors, perceived control, and self-esteem. Health Psychol 24(2):143–152

81. Ware JE Jr, Manning WG Jr, Duan N, Wells KB, Newhouse JP (1984) Health status and the use of outpatient mental health services. Am Psychol 39(10):1090–1100

82. Mishel MH (1981) The measurement of uncertainty in illness. Nurs Res 30(5):258–263

83. Schulman-Green D, Ercolano E, Dowd M, Schwartz P, McCorkle R (2008) Quality of life among women after surgery for ovarian cancer. Palliat Support Care 6(3):239–247

84. Holzner B, Kemmler G, Meraner V, Maislinger A, Kopp M, Bodner T et al (2003) Fatigue in ovarian carcinoma patients: a neglected issue? Cancer 97(6):1564–1572

85. Smets EM, Garssen B, Bonke B, De Haes JC (1995) The multidimensional fatigue inventory (MFI) psychometric qualities of an instrument to assess fatigue. J Psychosom Res 39(3): 315–325

86. Zimet GD, Powell SS, Farley GK, Werkman S, Berkoff KA (1990) Psychometric characteristics of the multidimensional scale of perceived social support. J Pers Assess 55(3–4):610–617

87. Havekes B, van der Klaauw AA, Hoftijzer HC, Jansen JC, van der Mey AG, Vriends AH et al (2008) Reduced quality of life in patients with head-and-neck paragangliomas. Eur J Endocrinol 158(2):247–253

88. Chelune GJ, Heaton RK, Lehman RA (1986) Neuropsychological and personality correlates of patients' complaints of disability. In: Gerald Goldstein RET (ed) Advances in clinical neuropsychology. Plenum Press, New York

89. Nyenhuis DL, Yamamoto C, Luchetta T, Terrien A, Parmentier A (1999) Adult and geriatric normative data and validation of the profile of mood states. J Clin Psychol 55(1):79–86

90. Trask PC, Paterson AG, Wang C, Hayasaka S, Milliron KJ, Blumberg LR et al (2001) Cancer-specific worry interference in women attending a breast and ovarian cancer risk evaluation program: impact on emotional distress and health functioning. Psychooncology 10(5): 349–360

91. Andresen EM, Rothenberg BM, Kaplan RM (1998) Performance of a self-administered mailed version of the quality of well-being (QWB-SA) questionnaire among older adults. Med Care 36(9):1349–1360

92. Pyne JM, Sieber WJ, David K, Kaplan RM, Hyman Rapaport M, Keith Williams D (2003) Use of the quality of well-being self-administered version (QWB-SA) in assessing health-related quality of life in depressed patients. J Affect Disord 76(1–3):237–247

93. Vacek PM, Winstead-Fry P, Secker-Walker RH, Hooper GJ, Plante DA (2003) Factors influencing quality of life in breast cancer survivors. Qual Life Res 12(5):527–537

94. Agra Y, Badia X (1998) Spanish version of the Rotterdam symptom check list: cross-cultural adaptation and preliminary validity in a sample of terminal cancer patients. Psychooncology 7(3):229–239

95. Fortner BV, Houts AC, Schwartzberg LS (2006) A prospective investigation of chemotherapy-induced neutropenia and quality of life. J Support Oncol 4(9):472–478

96. Bergner M, Bobbitt RA, Carter WB, Gilson BS (1981) The sickness impact profile: development and final revision of a health status measure. Med Care 19(8):787–805

97. Goedendorp MM, Gielissen MF, Verhagen CA, Peters ME, Bleijenberg G (2008) Severe fatigue and related factors in cancer patients before the initiation of treatment. Br J Cancer 99(9):1408–1414

98. Spielberger CD, Gorsuch RL, Lushene PR, Vagg PR, Jacobs AG (1983) Manual for the state-trait anxiety inventory (Form Y). Consulting Psychologists Press, Inc., Palo Alto, CA

99. Sukegawa A, Miyagi E, Asai-Sato M, Saji H, Sugiura K, Matsumura T et al (2008) Anxiety and prevalence of psychiatric disorders among patients awaiting surgery for suspected ovarian cancer. J Obstet Gynaecol Res 34(4):543–551

100. Den Oudsten BL, Van Heck GL, Van der Steeg AF, Roukema JA, De Vries J (2009) The WHOQOL-100 has good psychometric properties in breast cancer patients. J Clin Epidemiol 62(2):195–205

101. The WHOQOL Group (1998) The World Health Organization Quality of Life Assessment (WHOQOL): development and general psychometric properties. Soc Sci Med 46(12): 1569–1585

102. Schag CA, Ganz PA, Heinrich RL (1991) Cancer rehabilitation evaluation system-short form (CARES-SF). A cancer specific rehabilitation and quality of life instrument. Cancer 68(6): 1406–1413

103. Ringdal K, Ringdal GI, Kaasa S, Bjordal K, Wisloff F, Sundstrom S et al (1999) Assessing the consistency of psychometric properties of the HRQoL scales within the EORTC QLQ-C30 across populations by means of the Mokken scaling model. Qual Life Res 8(1–2):25–43

104. Ferrans CE, Powers MJ (1985) Quality of life index: development and psychometric properties. ANS Adv Nurs Sci 8(1):15–24

105. Ferrans CE, Powers MJ (1992) Psychometric assessment of the quality of life index. Res Nurs Health 15(1):29–38

106. Gupta D, Grutsch JF, Lis CG (2008) Patient satisfaction with quality of life as a prognostic indicator in ovarian cancer patients treated in an integrative treatment setting. J Soc Integr Oncol 6(3):98–104

107. Fox S (2004) Preliminary psychometric testing of the fox simple quality-of-life scale. J Neurosci Nurs 36(3):157–166

108. Kornblith AB, Thaler HT, Wong G, Vlamis V, Lepore JM, Loseth DB et al (1995) Quality of life of women with ovarian cancer. Gynecol Oncol 59(2):231–242

109. Lindley CM, Hirsch JD, O'Neill CV, Transau MC, Gilbert CS, Osterhaus JT (1992) Quality of life consequences of chemotherapy-induced emesis. Qual Life Res 1(5):331–340

110. Martin AR, Pearson JD, Cai B, Elmer M, Horgan K, Lindley C (2003) Assessing the impact of chemotherapy-induced nausea and vomiting on patients' daily lives: a modified version of the functional living index-emesis (FLIE) with 5-day recall. Support Care Cancer 11(8): 522–527

111. Coates A, Glasziou P, McNeil D (1990) On the receiving end – III. Measurement of quality of life during cancer chemotherapy. Ann Oncol 1(3):213–217

112. Crespi CM, Ganz PA, Petersen L, Castillo A, Caan B (2008) Refinement and psychometric evaluation of the impact of cancer scale. J Natl Cancer Inst 100(21):1530–1541

113. Downs KM, Wagner MK (1991) The development of an individualized quality of life scale for cancer patients. Presented at the Annual Meeting of the Southeastern Psychological Association New orleans LA, April, 1991

114. Downs KM, Wagner MK (1992) The individualized quality of life scale (IQOLS): psychometric properties and comparative population norms. Paper presented at the Annual Meeting of the Southeastern Psychological Association, knoxville, TN, march, 1992
115. Cleeland CS, Mendoza TR, Wang XS, Chou C, Harle MT, Morrissey M et al (2000) Assessing symptom distress in cancer patients: the M.D. Anderson symptom inventory. Cancer 89(7): 1634–1646
116. Portenoy RK, Thaler HT, Kornblith AB, Lepore JM, Friedlander-Klar H, Kiyasu E et al (1994) The memorial symptom assessment scale: an instrument for the evaluation of symptom prevalence, characteristics and distress. Eur J Cancer 30A(9):1326–1336
117. Northouse LFOR (1981) Questionnaire – patient version [cited June 17, 2009]. http://www.nursing.umich.edu/faculty/northouse/fearpt.pdf, http://www.nursing.umich.edu/faculty/northouse/fearscore.pdf
118. Mark TL, Fortner B, Johnson G (2008) Evaluation of a tablet PC technology to screen and educate oncology patients. Support Care Cancer 16(4):371–378
119. Padilla GV, Presant C, Grant MM, Metter G, Lipsett J, Heide F (1983) Quality of life index for patients with cancer. Res Nurs Health 6(3):117–126
120. Ferrell BR, Wisdom C, Wenzl C (1989) Quality of life as an outcome variable in the management of cancer pain. Cancer 63(11 suppl):2321–2327
121. Smith AB, Wright P, Selby P, Velikova G (2007) Measuring social difficulties in routine patient-centred assessment: a Rasch analysis of the social difficulties inventory. Qual Life Res 16(5):823–831

Index

Printing: Ten Brink, Meppel, The Netherlands
Binding: Stürtz, Würzburg, Germany